CW01116962

Geriatric Medicine

Geriatric Medicine

Edited by

W. FERGUSON ANDERSON, O.B.E., C.St.J., M.D., F.R.C.P.
David Cargill Professor of Geriatric Medicine,
University of Glasgow

T. G. JUDGE, M.B., F.R.C.P.
Consultant Physician in Geriatric Medicine, Stobhill Hospital, Glasgow;
Honorary Clinical Lecturer, Department of Geriatric Medicine,
University of Glasgow

1974

ACADEMIC PRESS: London and New York
A Subsidiary of Harcourt Brace Jovanovich, Publishers

ACADEMIC PRESS INC. (LONDON) LTD.
24/28 Oval Road,
London NW1

United States Edition Published by
ACADEMIC PRESS INC.
111 Fifth Avenue
New York, New York 10003

Copyright © 1974 by
ACADEMIC PRESS INC. (LONDON) LTD.

All Rights Reserved
No part of this book may be reproduced in any form by photostat, microfilm, or any other means, without written permission from the publishers

Library of Congress Catalog Card Number: 74-969
ISBN: 0-12-057250-8

Printed in Great Britain by
T. & A. Constable Ltd., Edinburgh

CONTRIBUTORS

G.F. ADAMS, Wakehurst House and Queen's University, Belfast, N. Ireland

A.J. AKHTAR, Geriatric Unit, Eastern General Hospital, Seafield Street, Edinburgh, EH6 7LN, Scotland

W.F. ANDERSON, University Department of Geriatric Medicine, Glasgow University, Glasgow, G12 8QQ, Scotland

C. BLAKEMORE, Department of Psychology, Cane Hill Hospital, Gouldson, Surrey, England

J.C. BROCKLEHURST, Department of Geriatric Medicine, University Hospital of South Manchester, Nell Lane, Manchester, M20 8LR, England

F.I. CAIRD, University Department of Geriatric Medicine, Glasgow University, Glasgow, G12 8QQ, Scotland

C. COHEN, Department of Geriatric Medicine, University of Dundee, Dundee, Scotland

N.R. COWAN, Department of Geriatric Medicine, Stobhill Hospital, Glasgow, G21 3UW, Scotland

J. DALL, Victoria Geriatric Unit, Mansionhouse Road, Langside, Glasgow, Scotland

I.W. DYMOCK, Department of Medicine, Withington Hospital, West Didsbury, Manchester, M20 8LR, England

A.N. EXTON-SMITH, Department of Geriatric Medicine, University College Hospital, London, England

IRIS I.J.M. GIBSON, Geriatric Unit, Southern General Hospital, Glasgow, G51 4TF, Scotland

ANNE J.J. GILMORE, University Department of Geriatric Medicine, University of Glasgow, Glasgow G12 8QQ, Scotland

M.F. GREEN, Department of Geriatric Medicine, The Royal Free
    Hospital, Gray's Inn Road, London, WC1X 8LF, England

M.R.P. HALL, Department of Geriatric Medicine, University of
    Southampton, Southampton, England

J.A. HUET, International Centre of Social Gerontology, Paris,
    France

B. ISAACS, Department of Geriatric Medicine, Royal Infirmary,
    Glasgow, Scotland

J.O. JOHNSTON, Social Work Department, Corporation of Glasgow,
    23 Montrose Street, Glasgow, G2, Scotland

T.G. JUDGE, Department of Geriatric Medicine, Stobhill Hospital,
    Glasgow, G21 3UW, Scotland

R.D. KENNEDY, Department of Geriatric Medicine, Stobhill
    Hospital, Glasgow, G21 3UW, Scotland

JANET McCALL, Geriatric/Psychiatric Division, Southern General
    Hospital, Glasgow G51 4TF, Scotland

R.A. ROBINSON, University Department of Psychiatry, Western
    General Hospital, Edinburgh, Scotland

J. WILLIAMSON, Department of Geriatric Medicine, University of
    Liverpool, Liverpool, England

T.S. WILSON, Department of Geriatric Medicine, Barncoose
    Hospital, Redruth, Cornwall, England

PREFACE

This book is an edited version of the papers given at an International Conference held in Glasgow in September, 1972. The speakers were selected for their specialist knowledge and the resultant text represents an up-to-date account of Geriatric Medicine.

We wish to thank Miss Irene Pearson for her untiring efforts to produce such a high quality print, and our publishers, Academic Press Ltd., for their help and enthusiasm.

November, 1973

W.F. ANDERSON
T.G. JUDGE

C O N T E N T S

ADVANCES IN EDUCATION: W. Ferguson Anderson	1
Techniques in teaching geriatric medicine: C. Cohen	9
Education in geriatric nursing: Janet McCall	19
Social workers' needs for education: J.O. Johnston	33
ADVANCES IN PSYCHOLOGY AND PSYCHIATRY: C. Blakemore	41
The role of drug therapy in geriatric psychiatry: R.A. Robinson	47
Depression: J. Williamson	67
Community surveys and mental health: Anne J.J. Gilmore	77
Environment and mental health: T.S. Wilson	95
Drugs and memory: T.G. Judge	107
ADVANCES IN TECHNIQUES OF DIAGNOSIS, TREATMENT AND RESEARCH: F.I. Caird	117
Recent advances in incontinence: J.C. Brocklehurst	123
New views on stroke: G.F. Adams	135
ADVANCES IN GERIATRIC MEDICINE: J. DALL	147
Endocrinology in the elderly: M.F. Green	153
Parkinsonism: F.I. Caird	171
Advances in the treatment of leukaemia: Iris I.J.M. Gibson	185

Progress in geriatric gastroenterology: I.W. Dymock	191
Recent advances in respiratory diseases: A.J. Akhtar	199
Recent advances in cardiology: R.D. Kennedy	213

ADVANCES IN NUTRITION AND SOCIOLOGY: B. Isaacs   225

Nutrition in the elderly: T.G. Judge	231
Vitamins and the elderly: A.N. Exton-Smith	247
Preventive aspects of geriatrics: N.R. Cowan	269
Social gerontology: J.A. Huet	283
Operational research and social need: M.R.P. Hall	293
The way ahead: W. Ferguson Anderson	307

Subject Index   317

ADVANCES IN EDUCATION

ADVANCES IN EDUCATION

Chairman's Remarks

WILLIAM FERGUSON ANDERSON
Professor in Geriatric Medicine
University of Glasgow

Geriatric medicine can be defined as the branch of general medicine concerned with the maintenance of health in old people and with the clinical, social, preventive and remedial aspects of illness in the elderly. This subject has become of increasing interest because of the larger numbers of older people in all developed societies, and because of the desire of the citizens in these countries to provide a comprehensive and meaningful service for older people.

The elderly individual requires much more provision of health and social service than is at present available, and large sums of money will require to be spent on the care of old people. To ensure the sympathetic and correct handling of the elderly with the aim of using the resources of each country to the best possible purpose, there is need for education. This educational process applies not only to medical students, doctors, members of the health team such as nurses, social workers and the para-medical staff, but also to the general public, and any country which sets up a geriatric service without supplying correct information to the public at large in what the service is aiming at will be faced with grave difficulties. One of the most important aspects of education in geriatric medicine is the endeavour to convey to the man in the street the aims and objectives of such a system. People tend to look upon doctors particularly interested in the elderly as if such physicians have one endeavour only, that is to prolong life, no matter the quality for as long as possible. While no physician interested in old people would ever wish to end an elderly individual's life, the main aim of any service for old people is to enable the elderly citizens to live as long as is possible in an optimum state of health. The endeavour then is to improve the quality of life, to make certain that older people live, if possible, in their own homes in as happy and as healthy a state as can be.

Training in the subject of geriatric medicine must be introduced into the undergraduate teaching of medical students. It can be stated that apart from paediatricians and obstetricians most future doctors will largely be concerned with older people and their problems.

During the medical student's undergraduate training, instruction in the anatomical, physiological and psychological changes associated with ageing should be given and this is best done in the earlier years of training. At the same time insight into future epidemiological trends and to the social needs of older people must also be included.

The existing work pattern of everyday life should be stated and the difficulties associated with retirement, housing and income during retirement should be explained.

From experience in Glasgow this type of approach is welcomed by the medical student who is most interested in the total care of his individual patient. When hospital classes commence and the medical student begins clinical studies, the special symptomatology of disease in old people must be taught; the unreliability of pain as a symptom, the common upset of postural control, the altered response to environmental temperature change, with the frequent absence of fever in acute illness, and the dulling of the sensation of thirst, are points to be noted. This teaching will include certain principles, multiple pathology is the rule rather than the exception with the older patient, the onset of disease is frequently insidious and the quiet and atypical presentation of a common illness is much more frequently seen than a rare disease. It can be explained also that elderly people often make an unexpectedly complete recovery and that prognosis in the elderly is a subject of extreme difficulty.

The student may well have noted from his experience of everyday life the existence of an élite of the elderly and the fact that many older people come into hospital with their first illness in advanced old age. The medical student should also be encouraged to see the value of preventative geriatrics, of endeavouring to pick up illness at the earliest point in the course of the disease, often before the older person has realised that he or she is ill. The concept of the self-reporting of illness to the doctor, so commonly correct in younger age groups, is not applicable to people in advanced age. These individuals are very frequently unable to distinguish symptoms which they attribute to ageing from those which in fact are due to disease.

It is important also to encourage the medical student to visit ill old people in their own homes and this is best done in company with a physician trained in geriatric medicine.

The training of the specialist in geriatric medicine initially follows the same course as that of a general physician. It is useful to allow the young doctor to spend six months in an acute geriatric assessment unit in a teaching hospital immediately after qualifying if he so desires, as many physicians are thus attracted to this speciality. After this phase, however, the doctor is encouraged to go away from geriatric medicine and train as a general physician, and after this training to return to complete his postgraduate instruction at pre-consultant status (senior registrar level) and spend two years in the geriatric service.

During these two years the use of the assessment unit in diagnosis, the value of continuing care of people by follow-up on discharge, the link between the hospital and the health centre, the provision of services by the social work department and the immense and unremitting value of the general practitioner to the old person, are essential components of his instruction. The physician in geriatric medicine takes part in pre-retirement training courses, lectures to those who have retired, and gives courses of instruction to all those engaged in statutory or voluntary services for the elderly.

The physicians training in geriatrics are encouraged to spend time in the wards of the psychiatrist, to study rehabilitation, to become interested in neurology and in locomotor diseases. It is best if these doctors can find time to visit other centres in their own country and abroad to see the type of work being done there. In his final year of training an endeavour is made to initiate such a physician into research projects and to show him the vast amount of knowledge still to be obtained in this discipline.

It can never be said that training in geriatric medicine is required only for medical students and physicians. The nurse and social worker have an essential part to play in health care schemes as have the physiotherapist, occupational therapist, speech therapist and chiropodist. All these professional individuals require interest and stimulation in this exciting subject. The value which they have in their individual care of older people must be demonstrated to them and the immense help which they can give to the elderly individual must be shown.

If there was an adequate pay structure for physiotherapists, occupational therapist, speech therapist and chiropodists, it is certain there would be no shortage, as experience has shown that younger people in particular are immensely interested in older people and can see ways of helping them often new and not revealed to those in the older age range. It is just not true to say that young people are not interested in learning of the difficulties of older citizens provided that the amenity for teaching is adequate and the circumstances of instruction good.

TECHNIQUES IN TEACHING GERIATRIC MEDICINE

CYRIL COHEN

Honorary Senior Lecturer
Department of Geriatrics
University of Dundee

The objectives of any project should be defined before the techniques which can be used to achieve these objectives are described. In geriatric medicine, the most important task is still the need to alter the attitude which people have to old age.

Elderly people themselves often think that when they become old and ill, little can be done to help them, and they may say "what can I expect at my age, doctor?" Unfortunately their relatives may share this opinion, and some professional people with whom they come in contact do little to dispel this viewpoint.

The principles of geriatric medicine are based on the fact that old age is not a disease, although the ageing process may make tissues more susceptible to disease. Diagnosis must precede treatment and prognosis, and the elderly person has the capacity to respond to a treatment programme. The four dimensions of geriatric medicine should be considered in every case - physical illness or disability, mental illness or reaction to physical illness, social problems and economic factors. Diagnosis must include assessment of disease and disability; treatment must include rehabilitation (of the four dimensions if necessary) and possibly resettlement. The importance of the needs of elderly people in long-term care in hospital or residential accommodation must also be emphasised.

The first technique to consider is the way in which those who are treating or caring for the elderly deal with their patients (or clients) and the interested relatives. The staff should create an atmosphere of optimism, the patients will require individual words of encouragement and relatives will require periodic progress reports and to be involved in discussions about the nature of future care for the patient. Some doctors prefer to discuss these details with individuals, others have experimented with clinics for groups of relatives. In some cases a demonstration by the patient and discussion with the physiotherapist and/or occupational therapist may dispel fears which the relatives have been harbouring.

There is, however, a need to supply this type of information to the public in general, and Professor Anderson has said elsewhere that he would like to see more use made of television and the radio for this purpose. He envisages a type of "Coronation Street" or "The Archers" programme which could include "geriatric information" in an informal setting.

In the county of Angus, my wife, who is co-vicechairman of the County Old People's Voluntary Welfare Committee, has initiated another technique in an attempt, amongst other things, to alter attitudes to old age. She is the editor of a magazine called Angus Account which is distributed free of charge to the elderly in the county via pensioners' clubs, the meals-on-wheels services, and a number of general practitioners. The printing costs are paid by the County Council and the magazine contains informative articles on nutrition, dietetics and health. The elderly readers are encouraged to contribute personal articles about yester-year, poems, anecdotes and a regular competition (with prizes) also attracts interest.

By these means helpful information and optimism can be transmitted both at a personal level and to groups of people.

Lecture Room Facilities

Figure 1 illustrates the technique which was used to create lecture room facilities within the same building which houses the Assessment Unit in one of the two teaching hospitals in Dundee.[1,2] The lecture theatre can also be used for physiotherapy classes for the patients, and equipment can easily be put to one side when lectures are being given. The proximity of the lecture room to the wards makes it more convenient to bring patients to the students for clinical demonstrations. This avoids the difficulties which occur with the traditional method of clinical teaching when a large number of students crowd round a hospital bed. There is a two-way communication system between the lecture room and the projection room and the latter is sound proofed. Nearby there is a comprehensive library of geriatric literature, a seminar room and the offices for the clinical staff.

Teaching Programme

Table 1 shows an example of the teaching programme for final year medical students. The students are now divided into three classes and each group attends for 2 hours each week throughout one academic term. A combination of lectures, tutorials, clinical demonstrations and discussions breaks the monotony of a comprehensive teaching programme. Each teaching method lasts no longer than 30 minutes and there is always a short break in each 2-hour period for a cup of tea or coffee.

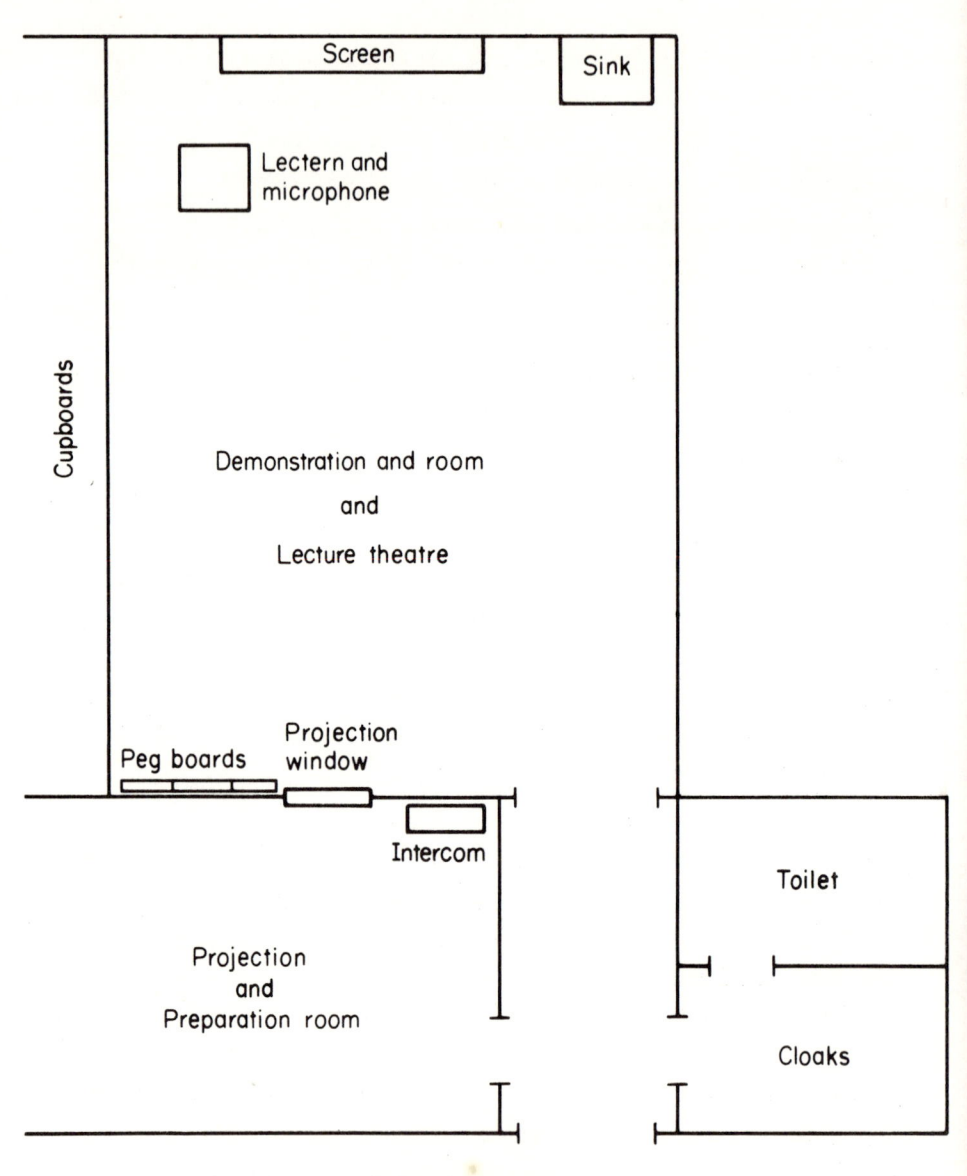

Geriatric teaching unit
Maryfield hospital, Dundee

Figure 1

Table 1

Spring Term 1968 - Final Year Medicine
Teaching Programme

Date				
Jan. 11th-13th	Introduction	Principles of rehabilitation	Clinical cases	Dangers of bed rest
Jan. 18th-20th	Demographic aspects	Practical aspects of rehabilitation		
Jan. 25th-27th	Principles of diagnosis	Clinical demonstration barriers to recovery		Fits, faints and falls
Feb. 1st-3rd	Heart disease in elderly	Clinical demonstration		Genito urinary problems in the elderly
Feb. 8th-10th	Terminal care	Clinical demonstration diabetes mellitus		Hypothermia
Feb. 15th-17th	Therapeutics	Clinical demonstration of locomotor disabilities		
Feb. 22nd-24th	Prescription of occupational therapy	Visit to the O.T. dept.	Clinical cases	Causes of disturbed behaviour
Feb. Mar. 29th-2nd	Tape recording speech disorder	Delirium Depression Dementia	Domiciliary Assessment Visits	
Mar. 7th-9th	Preventive geriatrics	Preparation for retirement	Postscript	

Teaching Methods

Table 2 shows the methods which have been evolved to make traditional teaching methods more attractive. Audio-visual aids have to be used with care, and the help of trained technicians in preparing wall charts, static demonstrations, colour slides, material for overhead projection, cine films, etc. is invaluable.

Slides for projection require careful preparation. Perhaps 8 lines of information should be the maximum for each slide and the letter size should be such that the lecturer should not have to say "I hope you can see this at the back of the hall". Judicious use of colour may make it possible to show the slides without fully darkening the lecture room. This avoids distraction during a lecture, when the main lights have to be put on and off intermittently. Horizontal letters on graphs and histograms makes them more readily appreciated and, of course, slides should be cleaned before projection.

The overhead projector is useful for someone who cannot draw clearly on a blackboard and tape recordings are helpful in illustrating problems of speech and changes in the voice in, for example, hypothyroidism, before and after treatment.

Experiments with video-tape recordings have been restricted because of the expense involved and closed-circuit television has not yet been installed.

The use of cine-film (and video-tape) has a special place in teaching geriatric medicine. The clinical picture of many conditions may continue for many months before a final result is achieved and students may not appreciate the steps in the patient's progress if they only see the patient once or twice during the course of diagnosis, treatment and rehabilitation. The full story can be telescoped in time by putting together serial cine films which have been taken before, during and after the treatment programme.

Table 2

Department of Geriatrics
University of Dundee

Teaching Methods

---

1. Tutorials.
2. Bedside teaching - physical signs, etc.
3. Practical demonstrations, e.g. physiotherapy, occupational therapy.
4. Clinical demonstrations - cases showing application of geriatric medicine to patient care.
5. Static demonstrations.
6. Audio visual aids:
    (1) wall charts and drawings
    (2) colour slides
    (3) overhead projection   } Teaching in Depth
    (4) tape recordings
    (5) serial cine films.
7. Video-tape recording.
8. Close-circuit television.

The technique of teaching in depth can be illustrated by the presentation of osteomalacia. A short tutorial with charts, slides and radiographs can be used to introduce the main points in history, symptomatology, investigations and pathology. Serial cine films will emphasise the associated myopathy and its response to treatment. If a patient can be presented in a clinical demonstration at the same time, an impressive contrast can be made between a treated and untreated case, and students are also reminded that patients are people and not just shadows on a film. Teaching in depth can also be illustrated with cases of hypothyroidism or cerebro-vascular disease with neurological barriers to rehabilitation. In addition to the above, tape recordings of voice or speech defects can be used and disabilities due to hemianopia or loss of spatial discrimination can be illustrated on film.

Teaching Commitments

Table 3 shows the teaching commitments of the staff in the Department of Geriatrics and, in addition to professional audiences, the importance of lecturing to non-medical audiences is emphasised. This is an important way in which an attempt can be made to alter attitudes to old age. The members of women's guilds, rural institutes, Red Cross, round table, rotary, etc., often ask for talks on the care of the elderly and this degree of interest perhaps makes the task easier.

The Lecturer

In all these endeavours to disseminate information about geriatric medicine, the lecturer is an important person, and he should be aware of the techniques which may help in the presentation of his case. Only brief comment can now be made.

Audiences may be distracted if the lecturer wanders about the platform, jingling money in his pocket, fiddling with a piece of chalk or a pointer or saying "umm" too frequently. Equally

Table 3

Department of Geriatrics
Maryfield Hospital, Dundee

TEACHING COMMITMENTS

1. Undergraduates (a) 4th and 5th year students - clinical medicine.
   (b) Final year students - geriatric medicine.

2. Postgraduates: (a) General Practitioner Refresher courses.
   (b) Junior Staff in-service training.
   (c) D.P.H. Students.

3. Pupil nurses and student nurses training programmes.

4. Health visitors.

5. District nurses.

6. Lectures to various non-medical audiences.

disconcerting may be the lecturer who remains bonded to the lectern throughout his talk which he may be tempted to read, and so present a view of the top of his forehead for anything up to 45 minutes. Eye contact with the audience enhances the presentation. For those who need spectacles in order to read their notes, "half lenses" obviates the temptation for the lecturer to keep taking off and putting on his spectacles which may also create a distraction.

A lecturer may obtain help from his colleagues (or a long-suffering wife) if they are asked to evaluate the technique which he has developed and which he should be prepared to modify.

Feed-back information from audiences and colleagues allows a constant reappraisal of both the individual lecturer's technique and of the programme which he presents. Geriatric Medicine continues to be an important subject as the proportion of elderly people in the populations of the world continues to increase. Those who wish to inform people about this subject must constantly re-assess the quality of the techniques which they use in this fascinating subject.

References

1 Brown, O. Taylor (1969). Teaching geriatrics. 8th International Congress of Gerontology. Washington, U.S.A.
2 Cohen, C. (1968). Teaching geriatrics. Geront. clin., 10, 108.

EDUCATION IN GERIATRIC NURSING

JANET McCALL

Principal Nursing Officer
Geriatric/Psychiatric Division
Southern General Hospital

In the Hospital Advisory Service Second Report (England and Wales) 1972, it stated that it is rare to find effective nurse education in Geriatrics. Perhaps this is not surprising when we consider the evolution of our Health Services. We have suffered from the legacy of cultural and social attitudes whose roots are deep in history.

We have been training nurses for just over 100 years and this training was traditionally orientated to acute hospital care. The profession has however, almost continuously attempted to change and adapt its training to meet changing needs, and these needs are today seen as being met by a comprehensive type of training. That is, a basic education and training in the art of nursing of all age groups. This embraces hospital and community care, acute, preventive and long-term work, rehabilitation, physical and mental illness.

Specialisation is tending to be done on a post-registration basis, and this trend will undoubtedly increase in the future.

In fact, in the revised scheme of training for the Register, this concept has been recognised in that the nurse is now encouraged to think seriously about her choice of speciality for the last six months of her ward experience.

We are at present waiting for the publication of the Brigg's Report - the report of a committee which has been considering the future role and future training requirements of the nurse. It is not too difficult to guess that it will advocate the separation of the educational requirements of the nurse and the service needs of the hospital - every committee which has considered nurse education since the 1930's has advocated this. I sincerely hope they will state the other very obvious requirement and so make good the glaring omission in the training of the student nurse at present - that is experience and formal teaching in geriatric and long-term nursing.

At present in Scotland four weeks' geriatric nursing experience may be given as part of general medical experience, but few training schools in fact take advantage of this. The present General Nursing Council syllabus for the wider basic training does in fact state that this experience should be given. The Council confines this recommendation, however, to acute assessment wards, the logic of which is obscure as it hardly gives comprehensive experience in geriatric care.

However, in some measure, we can at present give our student nurses experience in this field if we so desire. All areas, however, used for nurse training must be approved by the G.N.C., and approval is granted on the basis of experience available, the facilities available, e.g. bed spacing, equipment, the number of toilets and baths, etc., the staff/patient ratios, and the number of trained staff available for teaching the students. If we cannot meet these requirements satisfactorily, we cannot give our students this valuable experience.

In nursing, as we know so well, standards of care and teaching are closely related to environment. It has been shown repeatedly by various studies that if conditions are suitable and planned to meet the needs of nurses, then the needs of patients are met. But even prior to the findings of the Scottish Hospital Centre planning team and Doreen Norton's research work, Florence Nightingale enunciated the truth that bad sanitary, bad architectural and bad administrative arrangements often makes it impossible to nurse.

In a recent report on geriatric medicine the Royal College of Physicians makes the point that there is great satisfaction to be had in the specialty of geriatric medicine. The report goes on to state that if this can be demonstrated to undergraduate and post-graduate students there is no doubt that the problem of recruitment into the specialty will be solved.

I am quite certain that the introduction of a controlled programme of training and experience for student nurses would have a similar effect in nurse recruitment into the field. Where this experience is at present given, student nurses have demonstrated a keen interest and their project work has revealed insight and an imaginative approach in dealing with problems.

If we do not offer this experience to the students we are denying the value, interest, and challenge of meeting the special needs of the elderly. We do so at our peril, for those attitudes, as we know so well, are quickly reflected in the attitudes of the students and so develop to become the attitudes of qualified staff.

Pupil nurses have for a long time had the advantage over the students of receiving formal training and experience in geriatric nursing. The establishment of this grade grew out of the recognition that formal training was essential for the large group of unqualified staff who were working in hospitals for the chronic sick. All their training and experience therefore, took place in the long-stay hospital. It was not long, however, before the acute hospitals recognised the value of the enrolled nurse and by 1967 one-fifth of all enrolled nurses working in hospitals were employed in acute hospitals.

Gradually teaching hospitals began to train their own pupil nurses, and so the experience offered to them increased in range.

26 weeks' experience in chronic sick nursing remains a statutory requirement, but there are signs that this will change as the training becomes more comprehensive in nature.

It may well be that in future pupil nurses will receive a 1-year's course in basic nursing with additional specialist experience after enrolment, i.e. geriatrics would be a specialty and would be taken as a post-basic course. Some experience in psycho-geriatrics will undoubtedly be included.

In Glasgow at present we have two post-basic courses in geriatric nursing, and in November a third one is being held here at the Southern General Hospital. These courses will all be run twice per year, and are for both registered and enrolled nurses. They are short courses and include no ward experience and of course receive no statutory recognition.

The recently formed Committee for Clinical Nursing Studies will in future be responsible for all post-basic training and education for the purpose of ensuring that courses are in fact effective and not used as a means of staffing.

The three geriatric courses mentioned are in fact for external students who are seconded from their individual hospitals.

Unfortunately the creation of the roll failed to meet the growing demands for increased numbers of trained staff. In fact, the large number of unqualified staff not only remains in the long-stay hospitals, but now exists in the acute hospitals, who could not survive without their services.

We were again faced with training this group of auxiliary personnel and it is only a matter of time before this training becomes formalised and more uniform. At present only guidelines on their duties are issued by the Home and Health Department and each hospital has its own training programme.

It is absolutely vital that training for nursing auxiliaries is carefully planned - that it is a continuous process throughout their service.

The practice of leaving untrained personnel to their own unassisted genius in caring for the sick was deprecated by Florence Nightingale, who saw no place for kind hearts and willing hands if they were not trained hearts and hands. "Terrible is the injury" she wrote "which has followed to the sick from such wild notions!"

Fortunately these wild notions which persisted for too long in the long-term field are now fading fast.

When using different grades of staff there is a dangerous temptation to divide tasks out into neat separate parts and to train staff in specific procedures. The overriding responsibility of the trained nurse must always be to assess a patient's total needs and to organise how best these needs must be met at any given time.

Often the most basic physical care in a certain situation demands the skill of the trained nurse - a frightened apprehensive patient, the patient in pain, the breathless patient, a patient who requires detailed unobtrusive observation, etc.

Nearly all basic nursing procedures are simple and can be delegated to suitable training supportive staff, in carefully assessed situations.

The art of nursing, however, as opposed to the tasks on nursing is not simple, involving as it does, clinical knowledge, observation, assessment, judgment, skill in relationships, and communication, and knowledge and understanding of human behaviour.

A bed bath may therefore one day be rightly the proper task of the qualified nurse, and another that of the nursing auxiliary - the decision being wholly dependent on the continuing assessment of patients' needs by the qualified staff. Training of staff in assessment of patients' needs and the difficult art of delegation is vital.

Another form of training required - not only in geriatrics - but in all fields of nursing is nursing research. Research applied to nursing I had never heard of until I became involved in geriatrics, and in purely clinical research geriatric nursing certainly leads the field. Doreen Norton pioneered clinical nursing research and the value of her work in practical terms is difficult to measure.

In Britain we now boast of two Nursing Research Fellows in Geriatrics, one in Manchester and one in Glasgow, and their work must influence future care of patients in all fields of nursing.

Other than in the field of obstetrics and teaching, the concept of systematic and progressive training for the qualified nurse is given scant recognition. There are signs, however, that there is a growing awareness of the need for post-basic study of clinical subjects.

Management training is now available for all Senior Nursing staff on a Regional basis and Study Days in clinical subjects can now more easily be arranged by Nursing Officers to meet the need of their own specialised units. Hospitals are now much less insular and accept wider responsibilities for the continuing education of the nurse.

The Victoria Infirmary has for several years now been running short post-basic courses for enrolled nurses - courses which have proved most interesting and popular, and the number of applications from hospitals and community reflect the need felt by staff for this type of continuing education.

The Royal College of Nursing in response to pleas from both the medical and nursing professions have been running courses in geriatric nursing for the past few years, and the University of London now offer geriatric nursing as an option for Part B of their Diploma in Nursing.

To close it might be interesting to you to hear of our practical training programme in current use in our Geriatric Unit for pupil nurses (Appendix 1).

We are very much against the principle of learning by sitting next to "Nellie". Each pupil is given a copy of our Geriatric Training plan in which the objectives of our training are clearly stated. Listed are various aspects of geriatric work in which she will be given experience. We aim to teach our nurses not only basic skills, but how to apply them with judgement according to the needs of the patient. The pupils are required to submit nursing case studies.

The Senior Nursing Officer and the Nursing Officers control this programme and guide and supervise the trainees, and evaluate the effectiveness of our programme. In addition, a Clinical Instructor teaches procedures in the clinical situation. The Ward Sisters are very aware of their teaching function as was demonstrated recently in their ready participation in a recently established post-basic course in geriatric nursing. This is as it should be.

It is vitally important that the special needs of the elderly are understood by staff working in all units - including acute general medicine and surgical wards.

Geriatric nursing is not so much a specialist branch of nursing as an acquisition of skills in dealing with this age group - an understanding of the special physical and psychological needs and the need for the support and guidance of relatives and a knowledge of after care and supportive services. It is analagous in this sense to paediatric nursing. The whole of nurse training might be regarded as a project - the care of the patient. All staff of all grades are involved in different depths and in Geriatric Nursing we must ensure that we provide:

(a) basic training for nursing auxiliaries, with follow-up lectures and demonstrations;

(b) active formal follow-up programme of clinical teaching for pupils and students in addition to formal lectures arranged by the School of Nursing;

(c) orientation programmes for new staff;

(d) in-service training for qualified staff in way of study days;

(e) refresher courses - attendance at external courses.

In this way I hope we shall ensure that our training in Geriatric Nursing will be truly effective.

APPENDIX 1

Department of Geriatric Medicine
Geriatric Nursing - Pupil Nurse Training Programme

1. **Introduction to Geriatric Nursing**
    (i) The meaning of geriatrics - preventive work; assessment; rehabilitation and long care; community care; the size of the geriatric problem.

    (ii) The geriatric ward - patient's day geared to meet the individual needs at any particular time (these change). The pace of the work is different in Geriatrics. The importance of adjusting to meet these needs. Flexibility of programmes for patient care. Attitudes to the elderly Dangers of immobilisation and lack of mental stimulation.

    (iii) How to cope with:
    - (a) Confusion in the elderly
    - (b) Aphasia
    - (c) Paresis
    - (d) Incontinence
    - (e) Care of bowel and bladder
    - (f) Care of unconscious patient
    - (g) Prevention of pressure sores
    - (h) Insomnia
    - (i) Fluid balance. Importance of fluid intake.

    (iv) Uses of medical and nursing aids, e.g.
    - (a) Zimmer frames
    - (b) Tripods
    - (c) Calipers
    - (d) Roller frames
    - (e) Ambulifts

2. The Needs of the Geriatric Patient
   - (i) Physical, mental, emotional and spiritual requirements.
   - (ii) Retention of identity.
   - (iii) Maintenance and encouragement of independence as far as possible.
   - (iv) Clothing and aids for disability.

3. Rehabilitation
   - (i) Occupational therapy; recreational and diversional therapy.
   - (ii) Physiotherapy.
   - (iii) Speech therapy.

) Visit to Department. Talk by each profession.

   It is important to understand the rehabilitation and supportive programme so that this can be continued and encouraged at ward level at all times.

4. Introduction to Supporting Care Following Discharge
   - (i) Health Visitor.
   - (ii) Social Worker; Social problems of the elderly.
   - (iii) Home Help Services.
   - (iv) Welfare Services, for example, meals-on-wheels.
   - (v) Supply of medical aids where necessary.

   One week on district with District Nurse attached to hospital.

5. Project Work
   Two case histories to be submitted to Nursing Officer.

6. Mental Disorders in the Elderly
   Talks by Psychiatrist and Nursing Officer. Visit to Psycho-Geriatric Unit and Acute Psychiatric Unit.

7. Drugs in the Elderly
   Drug administration and recording;
   Control of drugs;
   Common drugs used in Geriatrics.
   Aperients and sedatives.

EDUCATION IN GERIATRIC NURSING

8. **Dietetic Problems of the Elderly (hospital and home)**
   Talk by Dietitian;
   ? Visit to Diet Kitchen.

9. **Medical Cases**
   Complete nursing care of:
   (a) Congestive Cardiac Failure.
   (b) Cerebral Vascular Accident.
   (c) Disseminated Sclerosis.
   (d) Parkinson's Disease.
   (e) Depression.
   Problems of diagnosis; multiple pathology; threshold of pain. Discussion of case histories and special aspects of geriatric care in wards – medical and nursing staff.

10. **Required Reading**
    All relevant articles in nursing press (weekly).
    'Patients as People', A.E. Clark-Kennedy:
       Chapter 17 (Rheumatoid Arthritis);
       Chapters 11, 13, 14 (Depression).
    'Medicine in its Human Setting', A.E. Clark-Kennedy:
       Chapters on:
    1. (Arterial Degeneration)
    2. (Vascular Accidents)
    3. (Disseminated Sclerosis)
    4. (Inoperable Cancer)
    5. (T.B. in adults)
    6. (Elderly Unfitness – Ulcer of the Stomach)
    7. (New growth)
    8. (Care of the Elderly) N.T. Report
    9. (Physiotherapy Helps Nursing T. Report)
    10. (Incontinence in Old People)
        Nursing Research in the Problem of Incontinence, Doreen Norton.

11. Recommended Reading
    (a) Home Care of the Elderly. Rcn., Q.U.D.N. and N.O.P.W.C.
    (b) Looking after Old People at Home. Doreen Norton.
    (c) An Investigation of Geriatric Nursing Problems in Hospital. Doreen Norton.
    (d) Care of the Elderly. Rcn.

EDUCATION IN GERIATRIC NURSING

Geriatric Unit Training Plan

WARD				
	Introduction to geriatric unit			
	Geriatric problem of today			
	Needs of the geriatric patient			
	Importance of mobility			
	Care of paralysed limbs			
	Care of the aphasic patient			
	Care of the unconscious patient			
	Confusion			
	Mental disorders in the elderly			
	Dietetic problems in hospital and home			
	Preventive work			
	Assessment			
	Rehabilitation			
	Available care on discharge			
	Community care			
	Uses of medical and nursing aids			
	Clothing and aids for disability			
	Occupational therapy - ward level			
	Recreational therapy - ward level			
	Physiotherapy - ward level			
	Chiropody			
	Speech therapy - ward level			
	Control of drugs			
	Drug administration and recording			
	Common drugs used in geriatrics			
	Administration of sedatives and aperients			
	Ward rounds			
NAME	Case conferences			
	Project work - 2 case histories			
Legend		Instructed	Experienced	Proficient

Objectives: (1) to give P.N. an understanding of the specific needs of the elderly, to develop the skills required to meet these needs, and to enable them to utilise these skills in different situations; (2) to give an appreciation of the size of the problem and a knowledge of the geriatric services available; (3) to give P.N. an insight into the psychological problems of the elderly; (4) to stimulate an awareness of relatives' problems and their need for support, and to develop skills to give this support.

SOCIAL WORKERS' NEEDS FOR EDUCATION

JAMES O. JOHNSTON

Director
Social Work Department
Corporation of Glasgow

Perhaps this seems a strange time to discuss social workers' education in geriatric work. Throughout Great Britain, recent years have seen the statutory abolition of local authority welfare services, which were very largely concerned with services for old people, and have merged the staffs of these services with those of other services into comprehensive departments of social work. These are in England and Wales called departments of social services, although I must say I find this title extremely difficult to understand, realising that these departments do not embrace such social services as health and education. This move has led to a general assumption that the work which these social work departments will do in the future will be only "generic" social work and to the fear that in this generalisation of work the needs of old people will be neglected This fear is certainly understandable, but in my view it is without much foundation.

I think it is important for all of us who are interested in the organisation and deployment of services to see exactly what it is that recent legislation has done. It has abolished statutory specialisation of social work services. It has done nothing at all to abolish or impede professional specialisation, that is, specialisation in areas of work and with groups of people selected from time to time by professional workers themselves. I think that specialisation of this kind should in fact be easier within the new organisation than it was in earlier organisations. The only qualification I would make to this is that it will take a little time. After all, the new organisations are very young. In Scotland they are less than three years old, and in England and Wales less than a year old. Inevitably, these organisations are taking some time to reform themselves and to work out their new structures and working relationships both internally and in relation to other organisations. Already in Scotland we can see regroupings of work beginning to happen, and I have no doubt that the same thing will happen before long in England, if it has not already done so. I believe therefore that in a quite short time new specialisms in social work will emerge within the comprehensive social work departments.

I do not wish to be interpreted as meaning that I think the new organisations will simply re-establish the former services for the old and handicapped as specialisms, with other specialisms in child care, probation and so on. What is likely to emerge is a new range of specialists relating to the needs of the work rather than to any statutory group. I cannot foresee in general at this stage what these specialisms are likely to be. The one question on which I expect you will wish me to express a view is whether one of those specialisms should be in geriatric work, and whether, if so, there is likely to be an early move in this direction.

My own view is that the answer to both of these questions is 'yes'. I think that work with the old is almost certain to be recognised as a field of social work which requires specialist study, and I think it likely that this will happen fairly soon. The reasons for this view are fairly obvious ones. The old form a very large proportion of the population, and also of the present total workload of social workers. The proportion of old people in the population has been growing for some time and is likely to go on growing in the foreseeable future. There is increasing public concern about the care and welfare of old people. The last point is one of considerable interest. I do not profess to know what are the reasons for this increase in public concern. It may be that people are in general becoming more humane, in some ways at least. It may be that the growing numbers of old people all have votes. It may be that with the import into this country in the last generation or so of substantial numbers of Asian peoples, their philosophies and cultures have rubbed off on us at least to this extent. Or it may be simply that all of us expect one day to be old ourselves - that we feel at some level "There *with* the grace of God go I". Whatever the reasons, it seems clear to me that there will be increasing demand for improvement as well as for extension of work with the elderly, and that this inevitably means some form of specialisation in their care and welfare.

I think therefore that this will happen fairly soon. I think also however that it would be unwise either to try to force this to happen, or to try to direct the processes from levels of authority. The new social work services will still take some time to work out the process of reorganisation and finding their feet, and they need time also to survey the whole battle from a new organisation vantage point. A second reason is that the new social work service has, at least in Scotland, powers which are much wider than, and very different from, those of the past. The effect of this is that the services do not need to think and act only in terms of old people, but can think and act before people become old, in ways which are likely to help to make old age better - however one defines better. The last reason for not hurrying the process of specialisation is that the whole educational and training system for social workers is being reviewed, following the appointment of a new statutory council to take charge of the process. The new council will also wish to have a thorough survey of the whole field before committing themselves to any important changes.

The development of a social work specialism in geriatric work will of course be concerned with specialised knowledge, approaches and techniques. I do not propose to talk today about any of these. For that purpose there are certainly better people than I, and probably better times than this. I would like to make a few comments about the base on which the necessary specialised knowledge and techniques should be built, and the context in which they could best be used.

I have no doubt that the initial training of social workers should be general and fairly wide in scope. I do not think I have to spell out the reasons for this opinion to an audience like this one, and I have perhaps only to ask the rhetorical question whether any of you would envisage that there should be geriatricians who are not first given a normal medical education. No doubt the same considerations would apply to the training of nurses. Again, much of social work practice is concerned with helping people to deal with changes in their living situations. Growing old is certainly change, and the basic attitudes which are relevant to that change are very similar to those which relate to any other major change - the attitudes which help the individual to adapt rather than give up, and to be able to learn how to adapt to change. To learn how to use change, rather than just to suffer it.

Again, it is important to sustain all the time the knowledge that the old are different from the rest of us only in some ways. In many more ways they are the same as everybody else. They have the same needs and the same rights for dignity of person, the self-respect and social respect, as everyone else and these needs and rights must be in the front of our minds all the time. Not special rights, just the same rights as everyone else. Again, in thinking about specialising in work with the old, we must all the time be conscious that very many of the difficulties of the old are caused in large part by poverty, unsuitable housing and difficulty in having and sustaining satisfying relationships with other people, and that these same afflictions are shared by the old with large numbers of people who are not old. We must remember that to some extent at least the relief of these afflictions can best be achieved by tackling the afflictions on a social scale as well as by focusing on the needs of the old. There is a risk by that specialising in the welfare of old people we might unwittingly lose sight of what can be achieved for old people in the more general context.

We in the social work services need to develop also special skills and aptitudes which will help old people in other ways. One of these is the skill of synthesising social work knowledge with other knowledge in ways which illuminate real needs and possibly ways of meeting them practically. It is highly dangerous for me to use medical analogies here, but I would like to take that risk in illustrating this point. Looking at the concentrations of population which we have today in cities in this country and in many others, I wonder what the state and form of health services would be like today in this country if doctors working a century ago had not been able to use their medical knowledge *and* much other knowledge to perceive public health measures which have substantially rid us in this country of such diseases as typhus, cholera and T.B. There is a real lesson in this for us in social work.

This leads me neatly to the last point which I want to make today. Here are some passages which I heard broadcast recently:

"I shall only mention four of the consequences of living in the condition of overcrowding and domestic discomfort. The first consequence is enormous liability to epidemic disease; to consumptive disease, and diseases of the lungs; and enormous mortality in young children in particular, partly of course from epidemic disease and partly from other kinds of disease which we know to be destructive of infantile life. The second consequence is that the sense of decency is injured inevitably, and ultimately is lost altogether. The third consequence is that almost inevitably a craving for alcoholic stimulents is generated, due to the want of what we may call natural stimulants, which go with us all to make up the idea of domestic comforts. It is the internal discomfort, it is the dreadful want of fresh air and of anything to relieve the monotony and dullness of life at home that drives many to the public house. The fourth consequence of this state of overcrowding, in badly constructed houses, is a great degree of moral degradation and of religious apathy.....

I am convinced that cleanliness, fresh air and the removal of overcrowded conditions of living could make typhus fever comparatively harmless.

While the causes of the mortality were probably in part atmospheric, the true sources of the excessive liability of Glasgow to such tides of disease and death are to be sought, not in these comparatively accidental circumstances, but in the permanently acting causes of high death rates and especially in the low standard of domestic comfort, the overcrowding, general squalor and physical degradation which are the unhappy characteristics of a large section of the population, and that these, again, are the direct results of permitting generation after generation to be brought up in houses of the worst construction, in which morality, decency and cleanliness are alike impossible.

There are eight points essential in a house: adequate cubic space; the means of separation and privacy for the sexes within the houses; a proper means of access; proper lighting and ventilation of rooms, as well as of lobbies; adequate privy accommodation; an adequate water supply; baths and wash-houses; airing and recreation ground".

These quotations are from a radio script written some months ago by a colleague of mine in the Glasgow Health Department and they are from the words of Dr. Gairdner, the first Medical Officer of Health in Glasgow, over 100 years ago. They were inspired speeches, which were short on statistics and validated research, but which were rich in rhetoric and passion and assertion. Their great value was that they made sense and could be understood and accepted by non-medical people in positions of authority and power. They were effective. Dr. Gairdner was an eminent academic and teacher, he said skilfully and confidently what he believed, and he used very tellingly the little factual evidence he had for his beliefs. He did this so well that action followed very quickly on his efforts.

With the other professional groups concerned with the elderly, social workers have to learn to communicate the practical essence of their knowledge and experience to those in authority, and if their main interest is in action rather than in just being right, they must learn not to be too inhibited in doing this by lack of absolute proof. This is not to undervalue research. It is to suggest that professional intuition based on research has its value also, and should be used.

ADVANCES IN PSYCHOLOGY AND PSYCHIATRY

ADVANCES IN PSYCHOLOGY AND PSYCHIATRY

Chairman's Remarks

COLIN BLAKEMORE

Principal Psychologist
Cane Hill Hospital, Gouldson

The past two decades have seen great advances in our understanding of psychological and psychiatric factors associated with old age. The importance of these advances has been threefold. Firstly, they have contributed extensively to our technique of diagnosis and treatment of the elderly, and hence they have provided the basis for an improvement in the quality of life experienced by the elderly. Secondly, developments in the fields of psychology and psychiatry have underlined the complex interaction between the elderly individual and his environment, and hence this has enabled us to realise the severity of certain social and community problems associated with the aged. Finally, our increasing awareness of psychological and psychiatric advances has contributed to our appreciation of these factors in research with the elderly, and hence they must exert an influence upon the actual nature of our research into the process of ageing and into the pathology of old age. Each of the five papers in this section of the Symposium contributes something to each of these primary areas; each has a specific emphasis on one area or another, but there is information and lessons to be learned in respect of each area from each of the five distinguished contributors.

The accelerating development of geriatric medicine will ensure that improvement will occur in the treatment, both medical and social, of the elderly section of our population. It is perhaps appropriate, therefore, that we should be careful to attend to the implications of our increasing knowledge of psychological and psychiatric factors on the design of future research. Much of current research in the geriatric field suffers from a lack of appreciation of the variables to be taken into account in the study of the elderly patient. Not infrequently investigations are carried out, involving perhaps a new drug or a new technique of social or environmental support, in which the effects of experimental variables are studied with patient samples which have been inadequately defined.

Anyone who has undertaken research in the geriatric field is aware of the difficulties encountered in defining the characteristics of the patients whom he wishes to study. We fully appreciate that the matching of patient samples is extremely difficult, if not impossible, because of the variation in the severity of disease or impairment of function which can occur in a sample of individuals whose homogenous characteristic is old age. For this reason we randomly allocate patients to every treatment group. But random allocation alone does not ensure that important factors will not operate to produce biases in response to those variables which we are investigating. Variations in mild degrees of depression may occur in certain difficult illnesses, but be absent with other forms of the illness, or memory may be invariably impaired in certain nutritional diseases which may themselves be more frequent in one or other section of the population. We may not wish to control our samples for factors of depression or memory in the particular investigation being undertaken, but knowledge of the possible influence of such variables should be kept in mind when designing the research. It may be of course that the best we can achieve is to ensure that the measure of their effect can be partialled out in the final analysis, but this is a considerable advance over the frequently occurring present state of failing to acknowledge their likely existence.

Finally, it must be said that if we are diligent in taking account of possible influential variables at the design stage of our research then not only would the quality be improved but also we may begin to have hard evidence of the importance of the early diagnosis of mild pathological states in the elderly. It is more than possible that the most influential advances in geriatric medicine are likely to be related to early diagnosis, and hence of increased scope for prophylactic treatment or environmental adjustment. I believe that the present five speakers have contributions to make in this respect from the standpoint of recent advances of psychology and psychiatry.

THE ROLE OF DRUG THERAPY IN GERIATRIC PSYCHIATRY

RONALD A. ROBINSON

Senior Lecturer
University Department of Psychiatry
Western General Hospital, Edinburgh

The vast proliferation of psycho-active drugs in recent years presents both a challenge and a temptation to a reviewer. With the increasing power and specificity of the armamentarium it would be possible to provide something like a therapeutic index.

But this is not the standpoint which I wish to take. It is rarely that a drug, or even a combination of drugs, provides a complete solution to a psychiatric problem. The remedy, particularly in the elderly, is likely to be physiological, psychological and sociological as much as pharmacological. Drugs are to be seen as complementing and not supplanting clinical and supporting skills.

That such an optimum prescription is not always achieved is well shown by Learoyd[11] who reviewed the admissions to a medical and psychogeriatric unit over a two-year period. He estimated that at least 20% had been precipitated by the adverse effects of psycho-active drugs. He is not alone in this experience. Many of us could testify that some of the most dramatic effects of drug therapy in the elderly are achieved not in initiation but in withdrawal.

A recent annotation in the Lancet[10] emphasised this growing problem of overdosage and intoxication. For these seems to be the trends if not the advances to which we have to direct our attention.

It is, of course, easy, from the safe haven of a Geriatric Unit, to criticise the prescribing habits of a non-specialist. A practitioner is in a difficult position. Unable to admit his patient to hospital, often unable to depend on proper supervision, he has sometimes no alternative but to attempt a chemical solution. Occasionally this will be successful; if it is to be successful consistently he will require better information about clinical psycho-pharmacology and a closer acquaintanceship with psychiatric skills and nosology.

It seems that if the aspirations for community based geriatrics and psychiatry are to be fully realised, the in-patient unit must be used more extensively and more energetically as a proving ground for new drugs and techniques.

In a recent valuable addition to the literature on psychotropic drugs,[12] Cole reviews some problems and methods peculiar to the geriatric psychiatric patient. The field in old age is both wider and more complex than with younger subjects. While drugs of proved efficacy will usually find their application in geriatrics, dosages and even indications can only be established by careful study in elderly populations. These patients are often unable to communicate adequately their symptoms or subjective states. Much of our information has to be inferred from their behaviour. We must, therefore, develop better methods of measuring and recording such phenomena. Physical illness can both complicate the clinical presentation and interfere with the absorption and effect of the drugs administered. There is much evidence to suggest that some older people tolerate or require substantially lower doses of conventional drugs than do their juniors.

Recent years have not seen the introduction of any novel drugs of generally accepted efficacy. The period has been rather, one of refinement and consolidation of our knowledge of known agents. A few drugs of proved worth have appeared in new forms, with the object of prolonging the duration of the effect, diminishing side effects, or reducing the frequency of administration.

It may be appropriate therefore at this point to review some principles of therapeutics. Few of us can hope to become expert with a wide range of drugs. It is essential to gain experience with one or two in each field and thus to be able to prescribe with confidence. It is now generally accepted that the "placebo effect" makes its contribution even where the drug is of proved potency. It is well to capitalise on this, once a therapeutic decision has been made, by prescribing with conviction and authority. Though it may have virtues in the scientific field, an attitude of cautious expectancy is not that which will commend itself to the distressed psychiatric patient.

It takes several years for the precise indications and side effects of a drug to be determined. If we succumb to the claims made for every new introduction, our knowledge will hardly advance.

Many drugs show a latent period before therapeutic effects appear. Patients and their relatives should be warned of this and of the possible appearance of side effects. A good example is the tricyclic anti-depressant. It is often helpful to explain that benefit may not occur for at least a week[16] and that in the meantime dryness of the mouth and constipation may well increase. Otherwise, since these are also symptoms of depression, the patient may lose heart and discontinue treatment.

The therapeutic goal must be evaluated carefully before commencing and the selected drug given over an adequate period before being replaced by another, if it is ineffective. It is seldom justifiable to multiply remedies in the search for an illusive response.

Treatment regimes should be reviewed regularly and superfluous drugs withdrawn - seldom abruptly. The tricyclics are again a good example. It is not unusual to find that a patient has been maintained on them for some years. Most depressive illnesses are self limiting; there is little evidence to suggest that the drugs protect against recurrence. They should in most cases be withdrawn gradually after three to six months.

Geriatric psychiatry presents its own special problems. Our aim as doctors is to make an accurate diagnosis and then to apply effective treatment. In general medicine our appraisal is based on signs and symptoms which themselves denote organic changes. These organic changes can often be demonstrated by pathological findings. In psychiatry our approach must be less "scientific". Pathological changes can be demonstrated less often and though our diagnosis too rests on the reading of signs and symptoms, their interpretation is more dependent on subjective impressions. "Symptomatic" treatments are our main weapons.

Geriatric psychiatry is a combination of general medicine and psychiatry. We have to use the tools, methods and medicaments of both. Our patients can first of all be divided into two main categories:

(1) Organic cases in which the symptomatology is predominantly of physical origin though its presentation may be "psychiatric" - demonstrated by behavioural or emotional disturbances.

(2) Functional illnesses which are essentially psychiatric but may have physical components. Among these are the effective illnesses and mania, depression, neuroses and paranoid states.

In the organic case the presenting feature is frequently confusion and restlessness.

It is important to remember that "confusion" is a sort of "common final path" arising from a variety of different causes. It is a descriptive term and not a diagnosis. It stands in somewhat similar relationship to the brain as does dyspnoea to the lung, and it would be as unscientific and impractical to seek one specific prescription for the confused patient as it would be for the breathless patient. The psychological precipitants may be fear, worry, failing memory, disorientation. On the physical side, toxic, metabolic and biochemical upsets or deficiency states may be implicated. These factors may be the basis of the psychiatric disturbance at any age, but homeostatic and adaptive mechanisms in the elderly bring their own special difficulties.

The subacute delirious state associated with infection, uraemia or electrolyte imbalance is frequently misdiagnosed and mishandled. Restlessness, mood changes or hallucinations are a frequent accompaniment of these conditions. If treated only with tranquillisers or anti-depressants the picture may quickly become unrecognisable and irreversible.

It is essential, therefore, in elderly people with psychiatric disorders to pay special attention to the physical state and to the investigation and treatment of abnormal findings. The case should be properly assessed in all its dimensions and a diagnosis made, before treatment can be commenced. However, it must be admitted that even if this is done meticulously, there still remains a small group of confused cases for which one can find no obvious cause. These then are the patients in whom it is permissible to treat confusion and restlessness symptomatically.

Sometimes, too, the severity of the disturbance demands more urgent handling. Disorganizing anxiety is a common feature in the presentation of acute psychiatric illness. There are few situations more distressing or anti-therapeutic than struggles with a frightened, confused and inadequately sedated elderly patient. Such confrontations can usually be avoided by prompt evaluation and action. Therefore if the upset is seen to be approaching crisis proportions it requires rapid and effective control. In my experience this is best achieved by the intramuscular use of a tranquilliser. Because of the hypotensive effect of these drugs and the possible aggravation of confusion by cerebral anoxaemia, the dose should not be excessive. Chlorpromazine (Largactil) 50 mgs. intramuscularly is usually sufficient. If it is not it can be repeated after an hour. Haloperidol (Serenace) 5 mgs. intramuscularly can be used in similar fashion. The respite gained gives an opportunity for analysis of the situation and the planning of the next step.

If the disturbance is less acute then the oral route is usually adequate. Diazepam (Valium) 5 mgs. or Sodium Amylobarbitone 200 mgs. are effective.

It has become customary, following the example of Hollister[7] to divide psychiatric drugs into the three major categories of anti-anxiety, anti-psychotic and anti-depressant agents. Though these indications are less precise in the elderly, the subdivision provides a convenient frame of reference.

In the account which follows I have for once followed my own advice and tried to confine myself to drugs of which I have personal experience.

Anti-anxiety Drugs

One suspects that the fundamental role which anxiety plays in many psychiatric pictures is not always fully appreciated. Thus suspicion, hypochondriasis and somatic complaints, hostility, belligerence, agitation and mood changes of varying degree may all have anxiety as their common substrate. The presentation will depend to a large extent on the preferred defence mechanisms of the individual. A knowledge of the life style and of the precipitants of the current problem is therefore helpful in deciding whether it is to be seen as a new development or is within the patient's habitual reaction pattern. In early organic brain disease, conflicts which have in the past been contained or suppressed are sometimes released in a sort of exaggeration or caricaturisation of previous personality traits. Sympathetic handling, reassurance and understanding are of course of prime importance, but the judicious use of drugs can aid the therapeutic process.

The benzodiazepines - Diazepam (Valium) 2-5 mgs. t.d.s., Chlordiazepoxide (Librium) 5-10 mgs. and Oxazepam (Serenid-D) 10-15 mgs. - have been shown to be more effective than barbiturates and all have been shown to be superior to placebo. The lower dosage level is usually adequate in the elderly; it should not be regularly exceeded in the presence of brain damage.

These drugs are all very similar in function, Diazepam being the most potent. However, the interaction of patient and doctor is probably the most important variable. Various studies have demonstrated the crucial effect of doctor warmth and enthusiasm.[19]

Hollister,[7] discussing the development of tolerance on repeated use and the withdrawal symptoms suffered by those who have become dependent on these drugs, points out that anxiety by its nature tends to be episodic. He suggests that brief courses should be used to relieve specific episodes. The fact that the patient knows that he can obtain relief may often sustain him adequately over non-drug periods.

The withdrawal reactions are of particular importance with this group of drugs and sedatives generally. Oswald[15] has shown in many studies the profound effect which prolonged administration has on cerebral physiology and the long-delayed return to normal functioning as reflected in E.E.G. studies.

Intravenous Diazepam has been found effective in status epilepticus,[17] and its use has recently been reported in acute drug-induced dystonic reactions.[9] It is often helpful in oral dosage in the control of drug-induced dyskinesia.

Meprobamate (Miltown) 400 mgs. and its analogue Tybamate (Benvil) 250 mgs. have fallen from favour in recent years though they have shown themselves to possess anti-anxiety activity. They are less potent than the Diazepines.

A new approach to the treatment of anxiety is the use of the beta adrenergic blocking agent Propranolol (Inderal) because of its action in reducing symptoms due to excessive adrenaline release. In general it seems to be more effective against somatic than psychological manifestations, though Wheatley[25] has reported a trial in which it compared favourably with Chlordiazepoxide. Some writers have suggested that this provides new support for the James-Lange theory of emotion, that visceral sensations determine psychic experiences.

An interesting application of the properties of Propranolol is reported by Eisdorfer.[4]

Eisdorfer starts with the idea that the decrement in performance on verbal learning tests with advancing age stems not solely from structural C.N.S. changes. Differences in scores may be related partly to a failure to respond when rapid response is required. Where the pace of learning tasks can be slowed, performance improves significantly. He suggests that the heightened and prolonged autonomic arousal found during learning task performance is directly related to the tendency of older persons to commit more errors. Propranolol by producing partial blockage of autonomic beta adrenergic receptor sites in peripheral and organs could be expected to modify most physiological components of C.N.S. arousal.

In the experimental design used, the administration of Propranolol 10 mgs. intravenously was found significantly to improve performance. The drug treated group made fewer errors both of commission and omission than did the placebo group.

Eisdorfer suggests that these results indicate that a state of heightened rather than depressed autonomic end organ arousal is responsible for the decrement of learning found in older age groups.

In concluding this section it is convenient to consider the sedative and hypnotic drugs. Barbiturates have been eschewed in the geriatric field because of their tendency to cause intoxication and confusion by cumulative effects. Such prohibition need not necessarily apply to the short acting barbiturates which as a night sedative have a time honoured role in the psychiatric hospital. MacDonald[13] concluded after a trial of Sodium Amylobarbitone 300 mgs. nocte on confused elderly females, that it neither improved nor aggravated their confusion. It is, of course, much cheaper than any of the newer introductions.

Amylobarbitone has been largely supplanted by Nitrazepam (Mogadon) 5 mgs. - another benzodiazepine - because of the absence of lethal effects in overdosage. However, where suicide is not a risk it would not appear to have advantage. Both are too potent for regular use in brain damaged patients. For them a milder hypnotic such as Dichloralphenazone (Welldorm) 1.3 gms. is usually adequate. For those restless patients whose confusion and disturbance is most marked in the early evening, a phenothiazine syrup such as Thioridazine (Melleril) 25-50 mgs. is often effective. And this conveniently brings me to the antipsychotic agents.

Anti-Psychotics

Most of our knowledge of these drugs has been derived from experience with chronic schizophrenics in psychiatric hospitals. This information is therefore of limited application in geriatric practice. However, there are some areas of common interest. Though their effectiveness in schizophrenia is established the mode of action is still not clear. Their benefits are due not simply to sedation.

A few years ago it was hoped that with growing experience "target symptoms" could be defined, for each of which a specific anti-psychotic would be pre-eminent. Thus aggressiveness, withdrawal and so on would each have its own special indication. However, such sanguine expectations have not been fully realised. Although seven groups of anti-psychotics, each with many members, are in use, we are perhaps fortunate that their range of activity can be encompassed in practice by a knowledge of three or four drugs.

The most widely used anti-psychotics are the phenothiazines and a butyrophenone. Chlorpromazine (Largactil) the parent phenothiazine is still the most generally useful, though its tendency to cause jaundice is a disadvantage, particularly in the aged. The incidence of jaundice has been estimated at between 0.5 and 1.5 per cent but has varied remarkably between different observers. The reaction is thought to be a hyper-sensitive reaction and is unrelated to dosage. Photo-toxic effects are also well known.

The piperazine derivatives, Trifluoperazine (Stelazine), Fluphenazine (Moditen) and Perphenazine (Fentazin) are in general more potent, are free from hepatotoxic drawbacks but are more prone to cause extra-pyramidal signs. Their "activating" effect – originally thought to be an advantage, when compared with the somewhat sedative effect of Chlorpromazine, is thought by some to be rather a "sub-clinical akathisia" which in its full development is a characteristic uncontrollable restlessness in which the patient paces up and down or moves constantly from one foot to another – the "dancing bear" syndrome.

Few of the phenothiazines are innocent of Parkinson side effects and this has been a serious limiting factor in their use in the elderly. Thioridazine (Melleril) with a piperidine side-chain has a lesser tendency to extra-pyramidal effects and has also some sedative action. It is, therefore, probably the drug of choice for the disturbed elderly patient. 12.5-50 mgs. t.d.s. conveniently administered as a syrup is usually adequate.

Haloperidol (Serenace) the butyrophenone, has already been mentioned in the control of the acute emergency. It has found an important role in the therapy of mania, but is worth a trial in the management of acutely disturbed behaviour of other aetiologies. If given orally a loading dose of 1.5 to 2.5 mgs. t.d.s. can soon be reduced to a maintenance level of 0.5 mgs. t.d.s. In my experience it has potent extra-pyramical effects and in the elderly should be reserved for episodic use. It is fairly free from sedative properties.

Most of these anti-psychotic drugs have also been advocated in low dosage as anti-anxiety agents. Thus Pericyazine (Neulactil), Oxypertine (Integrin), Trifluoperazine (Stelazine) are all useful in such circumstances and at this level of dosage are free from significant side effects.

I have come to believe that the sedative and tranquillising drugs should play only a limited and minor role in the treatment of the organic psychiatric case, at least in hospital practice. More important is the provision of a suitable milieu. This depends firstly on the surroundings, which should be as comfortable and non-institutional as possible. It depends also on "atmosphere" which should be permissive, supporting and non-threatening. We should attempt to adapt our ward routines to the needs and idiosyncrasies of our patients, and not the reverse. Fundamental to this is the understanding of the patient, the gaining of his confidence and the improvement of his morale and independence, particularly by occupational therapies.

A more specific use of phenothiazines in geriatrics is in the treatment of paranoid states and paraphrenia, that is, functional illnesses characterised by delusions and hallucinations occurring in the absence of intellectual impairment. Many of these illnesses can be controlled by the use of

Thioridazine or Trifluoperazine, though full insight is rarely
gained. A sort of "encapsulation" seems to occur. Post[18] suggests a starting dose of Thioridazine 100 mgs. daily increasing
at gradual intervals to 500 mgs. daily if necessary. If this is
unsuccessful, Trifluoperazine 10-20 mgs. can be tried with an
upper limit of 30 mgs. In my experience these higher doses are
likely to be attended by troublesome side effects unless the
patient is unusually fit and can be kept under regular supervision.

The question of whether to cover routinely these antipsychotic drugs with anti-parkinson agents is a vexed one. On the
one hand the incidence of extra-pyramidal effects and dystonic
reactions is high and on the other the anti-parkinson drugs themselves have their own anti-cholinergic toxic limitations. My own
policy is to give them only when neurological signs begin to
appear - a trace of cog-wheel rigidity or facial immobility.
Orphenadrine (Disipal) 50 mgs. b.d. (morning and mid-day) is
usually effective and seems less likely to give rise to toxic
confusional states. It has a "smoother" action than other antispasmodics and side effects in this dosage range are negligible.

In schizophrenia and paraphrenia drug therapy needs to be
maintained for an indefinite period. Lapses are the most frequent
cause of re-admission to mental hospital. "Drug holidays" are,
however, permissible and probably beneficial.

It is estimated that up to 40% of patients fail to take their
prescribed medication. This probably applies to both psychiatric
and medical drugs. As a result, the availability of the long-acting intramuscular depot phenothiazines - fluphenazine enanthate
and decanoate was hailed as a major advance. A great deal of
experience has now been gained in their use and "Modecate Clinics"
are an established feature of many psychiatric units. Though
their use in old age has not yet been fully evaluated, most
clinics include elderly patients among their clients and with

them the drug, particularly the decanoate (Modecate) has been found to be effective and reliable. The dosage schedule is too complex to give in detail, but ranges from 6.25 mgs. to 25 mgs. at intervals of two to four weeks. In the present state of our knowledge the induction period should be spent in hospital. There is good evidence that extra-pyramidal and dystonic reactions are most likely to occur within a day or two of the injection. The treatment should not, of course, be used in the presence of brain damage nor in those who have previously developed toxic reactions or Parkinsonism with oral phenothiazines.

Anti-depressants

I will leave the discussion of depression to Dr. Williamson, but some general comments may be offered.

The dichotomy, reactive or endogenous depression, seems to me to be of less relevance in the elderly. In general psychiatry too there seems to be growing acceptance of the notion of a continuum between the two. It is particularly the patient at the endogenous end of the spectrum who responds best to the tricyclic antidepressants. These drugs are worth a trial in any elderly person who, for the first time, develops frank depression in old age, whether or not there are clear environmental precipitants. The best response is obtained from those who present with the classical signs of early waking, duirnal variation, guilt feelings and loss of interest, appetite and weight. If anxiety or agitation are also present, an appropriate drug, e.g. Diazepam, should be used additionally until the tricyclic begins to exert its effect.

The many newer introductions in this field have not been shown to have any special advantage over Imipramine (Tofranil) or Amitriptyline (Tryptizol), both of which have rather similar pharmacological profiles, so the choice is largely a matter of personal preference. Amitriptyline is more sedative in its effect and is, therefore, to be preferred where a stimulant action is not desirable. There have been occasional reports of cardiovascular reactions with both drugs since their introduction. The low frequency of incidence of these should not deter one from their use if they are psychiatrically indicated.

Because of its sedative effects, many psychiatrists have prescribed the major dose of Amitriptyline at night; sometimes this has also avoided the need for an additional hypnotic. The introduction of Lentizol, a long-acting preparation, is thus a logical step. Reports by Haider[6] and Sims[24] both indicate that the new preparation is as effective as the parent drug. The equivalent doses used were Lentizol 25 mgs. nocte against Amitriptyline 10 mgs. t.i.d. and Lentizol 50 mgs. against Amitriptyline 25 mgs. t.i.d. This development is, therefore, welcome for the elderly, for the single bedtime dose is less likely to be overlooked.

In spite of the enthusiasm of some individuals, the hypertensive crises associated with Monoamine Oxidase Inhibitors present real dangers to the elderly if they are used in inadvertent combination with certain other drugs or foodstuffs rich in amines. The general tendency is, therefore, to use them only in exceptional circumstances. One of these is where there have been reactions to the anti-cholinergic effects of tricyclics, particularly retention of urine or in glaucoma. In such circumstances, Phenelzine (Nardil) 15 mgs. t.d.s. is worth a trial - an explanation of the dietary restrictions and a cautionary card should, of course, be given.

My own experience with Phenelzine in such cases has been encouraging. A recent study[20] showed that Monoamine Oxidase activity in hind brain, plasma and platelets increased with advancing age. Women had significantly higher values than men. These findings, correlating as they do with the observed clinical incidence of depression, raise interesting possibilities. Have we then been too conservative in our use of these inhibitors in the elderly?

A brief case history may help to underline some of these general observations and to indicate the complexities of psychopharmacology.

An elderly, well preserved woman had been maintained for many years on a benzodiazepine because of tension associated with her numerous life problems. At a point where her increasing difficulties seemed insoluble she became seriously depressed. Her practitioner substituted an antidepressant for the antianxiety drug. She was referred a few days later because of increasing agitation. It was believed that she required urgent admission to hospital because of worsening depression. Apart from her depressive symptoms, she complained bitterly of the "side-effects" of the new drug - ataxia, constipation and "intolerable tension". After evaluation it seemed likely that her somatic complaints had been greatly enhanced by withdrawal effects. During the course of a discussion of her problems, she was persuaded that the new drug would begin to function within a few days. Benzodiazepine was re-instituted in another form at lower dosage. She reported a week later that her acute symptoms had subsided within a few hours of beginning the combined medication. Within a month she felt "better than for years". Thus the practitioner's diagnosis of depression and the prescription had been correct, but the importance of explanation and of withdrawal reactions had been overlooked.

Lithium

The discovery of the mood regulating effect of Lithium was one of those serendipitous events which have characterised many of the great discoveries in medicine. Though reported by Cade[2] it has taken more than twenty years for it to achieve acceptance and respectability. Four main factors seem to have been

responsible for this tardy recognition. Some months before
Cade's paper appeared, Lithium salts had been released on the
American market as salt substitutes. Since these were mainly
used by sufferers from kidney or heart disease it was not surprising that there were numerous poisonings, some fatal. Within
a year or two the phenothiazines became available and were shown
to be effective in a wide range of psychiatric disorders, including mania. The interest of psychiatrists was then directed
to the exploration of the potentials of these apparently safer
and more promising drugs and, of course, later to the antidepressants. It cannot be ignored that since Lithium is a
naturally occurring product, not patentable, it did not have the
sales promotion which we have come to associate with other drugs.
Finally, mania is by its nature a difficult condition on which
to conduct double-blind trials. The enthusiasts for Lithium
therapy came to be regarded as a somewhat uncritical group.

The removal of Lithium from the restricted list of the
Food and Drug Administration only two years ago marked its
eventual but somewhat grudging acceptance. A detailed account
of the chequered history and indications for Lithium therapy is
given in an interesting monograph by Gattozzi.[5] The practical
management of treatment is covered in a paper by Schou et al.[23]
who have been one of the chief protagonists of the drug.

Lithium has been found to be most effective in mania, both
acute and recurrent, but there is convincing evidence that its
use can also eliminate or lessen depressive swings as well.[3] In
some depressed patients it appears to exert a prophylactic
effect.[14]

I am not aware of any report specifically devoted to its
use in old age, though most of the principal investigators have
included elderly people among their subjects. My own experience
is limited to its use in 15 people between the ages of 65 and 80.
All were suffering from recurrent manic depressive illness,

mostly of the bipolar type. Before commencing treatment we assured ourselves that blood urea and serum creatinine levels were normal and that the urine did not contain formed elements. Treatment was begun with 250 mgs. of Lithium carbonate twice daily, and serum Lithium estimations were made after one week. The dose was increased where necessary in steps of 250 mgs. at weekly intervals with the object of maintaining the serum Lithium at a level of between 0.6 and 1.0 mEq/l. When stabilisation had occurred the frequency of estimation was reduced to once fortnightly and later to once monthly. For out-patients, estimations and clinical re-assessment were conveniently done during day hospital or clinic attendance. A recent report of a double-blind trial by Hullin et al[8] describes a similar procedure. In the present state of our knowledge it would seem wise to initiate treatment in the elderly only under in-patient supervision.

Most of my own group of patients have now been maintained on the drug without untoward effects for more than three years. Though the results might not satisfy a critical statistician, I am satisfied that the treatment has made a useful contribution to the health and happiness of most of the participants.

Our most dramatic success was a woman of 70 who had been precipitated into a profound melancholia by the desertion of her husband. She did not respond to standard anti-depressant drugs and though temporary remissions were always achieved with E.C.T. she regularly relapsed within a few weeks. This sequence continued unchanged for many cycles. After the commencement of Lithium therapy she required only one further course of E.C.T. Since then for a period of nearly two years she has remained well, in good spirits and quite independent. She now lives alone, a considerable distance from the hospital, and cannot attend regularly. Blood samples are sent by post at specified intervals by her general practitioner who makes adjustments in dosage if these are indicated.

It must be stressed that the treatment has its dangers - though probably not more so than, for example, the insulin treatment of diabetes. Blood levels must be regularly monitored and patients and their relatives warned of the necessity for reporting side effects and of the potential hazards of electrolyte imbalance which may occur during intercurrent illness.

Other Drugs

Improvement in intellectual performance either on the basis of increased cerebral blood flow or of a direct neuronal effect has been claimed for many drugs. But the evidence from controlled trials is conflicting and efficacy far from proven. However, as I have hinted, the cerebral stimulants are not alone in the "suspected" category. A survey of the critical psychopharmacological literature demolishes many sacred cows.

The geriatric population explosion imposes on us an urgent need for study on carefully selected sub-groups of patients. Too often we proceed too hastily to larger trials where heterogeneity may confuse the issue. Many drug trials are performed on chronic populations where diagnosis is often difficult to define with precision and the possibility of significant response may be negligible. Interactive effects such as the stimulation and interest consequent on the administration of treatments and the assessment of response are further complicating factors. It is perhaps not surprising that in many trials placebo often seems as effective as drugs of proved potency.[21]

It may be that we have been too wide in our selection of patients or our instruments of measurement too crude. I will leave it to Dr. Judge to pass sentence!

A recent review of geriatric rating scales (Salzman et al.[22]) and a discussion of the measurement of mood (Aitken et al.[1]) may serve, hopefully, as useful stimuli for the sharpening of our tools.

References

1. Aitken, R.C.B. and Zealley, A.K. (1970). Measurement of mood. Brit. J. Hosp. Med., 4:2, 215.

2. Cade, J.F.J. (1949). Lithium salts in the treatment of psychotic excitement. Med. J. Aust., 36, 349.

3. Coppen, A., Noguera, R., Bailey, J., Burns, B.H., Swani, M.S., Hare, E.H., Gardner, R. and Maggs, R. (1971). Prophylactic lithium in affective disorders. Lancet, II, 275.

4. Eisdorfer, C., Nowlin, J. and Wilkie, F. (1970). Improvement of learning in the aged by modification of autonomic nervous system activity. Science, 170, 1327.

5. Gattozzi, A.A. Lithium in the treatment of mood disorders. National Clearinghouse for Mental Health Information. Publication No. 5033. (N.I.M.H. U.S.A.).

6. Haider I. (1972). A single daily dose of a new form of amitriptyline. Brit. J. Psychiat., 120, 521.

7. Hollister, L.E. (1969). Clinical use of psychotherapeutic drugs. Clin. Pharmacol. Ther., 10, 170.

8. Hullin, R.P., McDonald, R. and Allsopp, M.N.E. (1972). Prophylactic lithium in recurrent affective disorders. Lancet, 1, 1044.

9. Korczyn, A.D. and Goldberg, G.J. (1972). Intravenous diazepam in drug-induced dystonic reactions. Brit. J. Psychiat., 121, 75.

10. Leading Article (1972). Drugs and the elderly mind. Lancet, 2, 126.

11. Learoyd, B.M. (1972). Psychotropic drugs and the elderly patient. Med. J. Aust., I, 1131.

12. Levine, J., Schiele, B.C. and Bouthilet, L. (1971). Principles and problems in establishing the efficacy of psychotropic agents. Department of Health, Education and Welfare, U.S.A. Public Health Service Publication No. 2138.

13. McDonald, C., Mowbray, R.M. and Wilson, J.M.O. (1970). A sequential trial of amylobarbitone sodium. Geront. Clin., 12, 335.

14   Melia, P.I. (1970). A doubleblind trial in recurrent affective disorders. Brit. J. Psychiat, 116, 621.

15   Oswald, I. (1970). Dependence upon hypnotic and sedative drugs. Brit. J. Hosp. Med., 4:2, 168.

16   Oswald, I., Brezinova, V. and Dunleavy, D.L.F. (1972). On the slowness of action of tricyclic antidepressant drugs. Brit. J. Psychiat, 120, 673.

17   Parsonage, M.J. and Norris, J.W. (1967). Use of diazepam in treatment of severe convulsive status epilepticus. Brit. Med. J., 3, 85.

18   Post, F. (1970). The elderly paranoid patient. Recognition, diagnosis and treatment. Med. World 108, 2, 9.

19   Rickels, K., Lipman, R.S., Park, L.C., Covi, L., Uhlenhuth, E.H. and Mock, J.E. (1971). Drug, doctor warmth and clinic setting in the symptomatic response to minor tranquillizers. Psychopharmacologia (Berl.), 20, 120.

20   Robinson, D.S., Davis, J.M., Nies, A., Ravaris, C.I. and Sylwester, D. (1971). Relation of sex and ageing to monoamine oxidase activity of human brain, plasma and platelets. Arch. Gen. Psychiat., 24, 536.

21   Robinson, R.A. (1961). Some problems of clinical trials in elderly people. Geront. Clin., 3, 247.

22   Salzman, C., Kochansky, G.E. and Shaden, R.I. (1972). Rating scales for geriatric psychopharmacology - a review. Psychopharmacol. Bull. Vol. 8, No. 3.

23   Schon, M., Amdisen, A. and Baastrup, P.C. (1971). The practical management of lithium treatment. Brit. J. Hosp. Med., Vol. 6, No. 1, 53.

24   Sims, A.C.P. (1972). A sustained release form of amitriptyline. Brit. J. Psychiat., 120, 65.

25   Wheatley, D. (1969). Comparative effects of propranolol and chlordiazepoxide in anxiety states. Brit. J. Psychiat., 115, 1411.

DEPRESSION

JAMES WILLIAMSON

Professor of Geriatric Medicine
University of Liverpool

It may well be asked why a non-psychiatrist should be attempting to deal with a psychiatric topic. There are I think several justifications for this and I hope that, when I have finished, you may agree. In geriatric medicine we have succeeded more than in any other specialty in bridging the unfortunate and artificial gap between internal medicine and psychiatry. No one can successfully practise geriatric medicine without an appreciation of the fundamental importance of mental health, and without a good working knowledge of psychiatry. In addition, it is rare to find in old age a purely "psychiatric case" - in the great majority the psychiatric illness is only one of several disturbances of function associated with the multiple pathology and "vicious circles of pathology".[8] Thus many patients with depression present not with the symptoms of this illness, but with an aggravation of a pre-existing stroke, rheumatic complaint or heart or respiratory illness (or even with all these complaints simultaneously). Thus the Geriatric Physician may well see more cases of depression in the elderly than the psychiatrist. This was well demonstrated some years ago when I collaborated with psychiatrists in a trial of a tricyclic antidepressant in patients aged 65 and over. By the time the psychiatrist had entered six patients in the trial, we had mustered 40 (final diagnosis being made by the psychiatrist in all cases).

Definition of Depression

Depression means a disturbance of brain function as a result of which normal control of affect is lost. Mood is unrelievedly lowered and in addition there are in varying degree: (1) diminished power of mental concentration; (2) loss of physical and psychic energy and drive; and (3) characteristic sleep disturbance.

Many studies have shown that depression is commoner in the elderly and that most cases in old age are first attacks in previously healthy individuals, i.e., it is a true involutional melancholy. I do not propose to deal with manic depressive illness since it seems clear that this is a separate, genetically linked condition.[6,15] Manic depressives rarely present in geriatric practice in my experience.

Our own population studies in Edinburgh have shown that depressive illness occurred in 5.4% of a random sample of elderly persons (Maule, unpublished). Females showed a higher prevalence than males. These findings agree with other published studies.[2,7,12,14]

Can we give reasons why depression becomes commoner in old age? I think that several explanations can be advanced.

(1) Social Factors

There is no doubt that many old people in our society are lonely and isolated. Nearly a million elderly people in Britain live alone; two million draw supplementary benefit (which means they live just above subsistence level unless overtaken by inflation in which case they sink below it). Three hundred thousand old people have no inside W.C. or hot water. Seven out of ten live on the State pension alone. These are bare statistics but those of us who work in geriatrics know the human misery that lies behind them. For those who are not personally involved in geriatric work and who wish to gain an insight into the stresses and strains which afflict the elderly in our society, I can do no better than to recommend Dr. Isaacs' little book "Survival of the Unfittest".[5] The sense of alienation and not belonging which affects many old people is well known to us, and is perhaps now seen in its most acute form in old people living alone in multi-storey flats in our cities. Where environmental factors are adverse, reactive depression occurs and it seems likely that, if circumstances remain unfavourable for a prolonged period, a certain proportion of the sufferers will progress to a full blown depressive illness. It has been convincingly argued by Forrest[4] that the difference between reactive depression and "endogenous" depression is one of degree only.

(2) Psychological Factors

The psychological effect of loneliness and alienation is profound but it is likely that in addition more subtle factors are at work. Various studies have shown that there is an inverse relationship between the level of violence in a community and the incidence of depression and suicide. Suicide levels decrease in wartime, and recent studies from Northern Ireland have shown that in the strife-riven city of Belfast in 1969-70, the incidence of depression showed a significant decline.[10] This fall was most marked in the most violent areas of the city. The psychodynamic explanation of this is that if violent impulses cannot be "exteriorised", then the violence is turned inwards, resulting in depression and even suicide. It is easy to apply this argument to help to explain the rising incidence of depression in the elderly who have scant opportunity for "normal" release of aggression. They are gradually edged into a back seat in society, compulsorily retired at 60 or 65, their affairs are taken over by relatives and by protective state and local government officials. The common stereotype of contented old age is the silver-haired old lady sitting by a cosy fireside with all her comforts provided. In truth the "awkward" old lady who continues to battle with her neighbours, her family, the rent collector and everyone in sight may in fact be better psychologically adjusted. The same arguments apply to men who find themselves on the scrap-heap after retirement when they are expected instantly to assume a largely passive role.

(3) Physical Disease

The co-existence of disabling, painful, distressing (and sometimes humiliating) complaints based upon the multiple pathology of old age is depressing. I wish here to allude to the importance of the doctor's attitude to the patient with chronic illness. It can be argued that the negative attitude of most doctors to elderly patients with chronic disability can itself have a powerful depressing effect upon the patients. It has been suggested that suicide is in some instances precipitated after a visit to a doctor.[3] Put in another way, doctors tend to discriminate against patients who do not fit their image of "the patient everyone likes", i.e., the young or middle-aged person with reversible, preferably acute illness, who will be unendingly grateful and infinitely co-operative. (What about these advertisements for antidepressant drugs for patients of "previously good personality"!) That we continue to produce doctors who see their role as the management of such "ideal patients" is surely a damning indictment of present-day medical education.

(4) Biochemical Factors

There is in the brain a finely adjusted mechanism for the regulation of mood. It is reasonable to assume that, as with other control and homeostatic mechanisms, the ageing process has a deleterious effect and that the power to withstand stress is impaired in old age. It is well established that certain drugs can profoundly alter mood. Some of these drugs fortunately can be used to treat depression, while others may induce this condition, e.g. reserpine and methyl dopa which can be very dangerous in the elderly.

Animal experiments have shown that monoamine oxidase (MAO) levels increase with age in heart and brain in many species.[11] It has also been shown that the products of biogenic amine metabolism - 5 hydroxyindole-acetic acid (5-HIAA) and homovanillic acid (HVA) increase in concentration in the cerebrospinal fluid of elderly persons.[1] Similarly, Robinson et al.[13] showed that in the hindbrains of 55 persons dying from a variety of causes, MAO and 5-HIAA levels increased significantly with age. Noradrenaline levels on the other hand showed a significant fall. These observations, of course, fit in with the pharmacological effect of monoamine oxidase inhibitors and tricyclic drugs used as antidepressants. Both these series of drugs act by increasing amine levels in the brain - the former by reducing their enzymatic destruction and the latter by inhibiting their re-uptake.

Clinical Features of Depression in Old Age

I do not propose to discuss this aspect in any detail since the symptoms and signs of depression are well known. The cardinal feature is the lowered mood and impoverished psychic energy - the tense facial expression with vertical central furrows in the forehead often gives one the diagnosis even before the patient has spoken. Other almost constant features are the early waking, the morbid thought content and the loss of enjoyment of food (and other pleasures which ordinarily persist in old age). The elaborate delusions of unworthiness found in younger sufferers are rare in the elderly, although expressions of self-depreciation are common ("I'm being a nuisance, doctor", "I'm sorry to be wasting your time again", etc.)

Often in the elderly the depression is substantially or completely submerged in pre-existing disability. Thus the stroke patient having made satisfactory progress begins to fail to respond to further rehabilitation efforts; the rheumatoid who "goes off her feet". Most distressing of all perhaps is the patient who presents with a welter of hypochondrical complaints, eagerly claiming as her own any symptom proffered - note here my own negative attitude showing in the pejorative terms I have used to describe these unfortunates. Constipation is common and may lead to marked preoccupation with bowel function, to the intense annoyance and even disgust of relatives and other attendants.

I wish to mention one symptom which I believe to be associated with depression in the elderly and which I have not seen described. This is nocturia unaccompanied by urinary frequency by day. Where no other explanation can be found, it is important to consider depression as a cause and often justifiable to have a trial of antidepressant therapy.

Management of Depression in the Elderly

Dr. Robinson has already covered the subject of anti-depressant drug therapy. All I need say is that I have found tricyclic drugs to be safe and effective, provided the dose is carefully adjusted to individual needs. I do not hesitate to seek electropexy if drugs fail.

General management of the patient is all important and in this we attempt to apply rationally what we have learned about aetiological factors. The social factors is dealt with by mobilising social support - the family, neighbours - the impetus coming from the general practitioner and health visitor. At the in-patient stage, the occupational therapist and physiotherapist collaborate with nurses to increase the patient's state of arousal. This is later continued as a day patient. It is important to do everything possible to combat the psychological factor by involving the patient as much as possible in normal relationships with other people. Day centres and church activities ought to be of greater help here.

It is, of course, essential that associated disability must be dealt with as expertly as possible with restoration of maximum function and appropriate modification of environment and use of aids to living where appropriate. Dietary deficiencies must be attended to and often a course of vitamin supplements may be indicated where there has been a period of anorexia.

I wish to emphasise the importance of continued follow-up of elderly patients who have been successfully treated for depression. The chance of relapse is always present and it is quite illogical to expect the patient to seek help if it occurs. We know that old people are extraordinarily inept at self-reporting of illness and the very nature of depression makes non-reporting very probable - with diminished energy, desire not to intrude and be a nuisance, etc. Hence I would recommend that every old person who has had depression should be seen regularly thereafter by a doctor who is knowledgeable about this illness. I believe that effective supervision will eventually be possible by specially trained health visitors.

The Prevention of Depression in the Elderly

It would be out of character for me not to say something about preventive aspects since this has been my abiding interest.

From what I have said about predisposing factors, it is evident that depression ought to be at least partially preventable. In the field of primary or "true" prevention, we should aim at the alleviation of loneliness by better education, better retirement policies and retirement counselling, better social services and more rational and humane housing policies. We badly need new experiments in providing purposeful activity and recreation for old people.

In the field of tertiary prevention we can try to secure earlier diagnosis so that treatment will be more effective and the secondary effects of prolonged immobility and malnutrition may be minimised. Likewise, exhaustion and demoralisation of relatives will be reduced. Early diagnosis is largely a question of awareness of the kind of old person most prone to depression.

The Profile of the Elderly Person prone to Depression

(1) She is more likely to be female.
(2) She is more likely to be lonely or isolated.
(3) She is more likely to have associated painful, limiting and distressing illness, e.g., rheumatoid arthritis, Parkinsonism, stroke and illnesses associated with dyspnoea.
(4) She is more likely to have been recently bereaved, especially after a prolonged period of stress in caring for a dying spouse. The sudden loss of a sense of purpose, combined with the sense of personal loss and exhaustion is overwhelming. The bereavement, of course, may be the loss of an offspring ("Why could it not have been me, I've had my life").
(5) Recently rehoused.

It is possible now to speculate that in the future altered plasma levels of certain biogenic amines may assist in early detection of depression or even enable us to detect the pre-symptomatic stages. Then drugs could be used to correct the biochemical disturbance.

In our consultative clinic where we attempt to see and assess high risk categories of old people, we have shown[9] that 14% of attenders have depression. This is surely a remarkable yield of an eminently treatable condition.

I hope, therefore, that I have succeeded in convincing you that depression is common in old age, that it is often undiagnosed, that it is to some extent preventable. There are few conditions which have given me personally more satisfaction in diagnosis and treatment.

References

1. Bowers, M.B., Gerbode, F.A. (1968). Nature, 219, 1256.
2. Bremner, J. (1951). Acta Psychiat. Scand. Suppl. 62.
3. British Medical Journal (1969). Leading Article, 3, 61Q.
4. Forrest, A.D., Fraser, R.H. and Priest, R.G. (1965). Brit. J. Psychiat. 111, 472, 243.
5. Isaacs, B., Livingston, M. and Neville, Y. (1972). "Survival of the Unfittest", Routledge & Kegan Paul, London and Boston.
6. Kallman, F.J. (1950). Congn. Internat. Psychiat., 6, 177.
7. Kay, D.W.K., Beamish, P. and Roth, M. (1964). Brit. J. Psychiat., 110, 146.
8. Korenchevsky, V. (1961). "Physiological and Pathological Agency", S. Kangen, Basel.
9. Lowther, C.P., McLeod, R.D.M. and Williamson, J. (1970).
10. Lyons, H.A. (1972). B.M.J., 1, 342.
11. Nochmias, V.T. (1960). J. Neurochem., 6, 99.
12. Primrose, E.J.R. (1962). Psychological Illness. A Community Study. London.
13. Robinson, D.S., Nies, A., Davis, J.N., Bunney, W.E., Davis, J.M., Colburn, R.W., Bourne, H.R., Shaw, D.M. and Copper, A.J. (1972). Lancet, 1, 290.
14. Sheldon, J.H. (1948). The Social Medicine of Old Age. Published for the Trustees of the Nuffield Foundation, London.
15. Slater, Eliot (1938). Z. Ges. Neurol. Psychiat., 163, 1.

COMMUNITY SURVEYS AND MENTAL HEALTH

ANNE J.J. GILMORE

Lecturer in Geriatric Medicine
University of Glasgow

The purposes of mental health surveys are many and varied. The most usual purpose is that of establishing a prevalence rate for particular mental disorders in order to assess the size of the problem within the community studied. It may be argued that this is best done in community research since those retrospective studies which concentrate on admission to an institution give little indication of the prevalence of the disorders in the community at large. Admission to any institution, especially a geriatric one, is usually the result of a combination of medical, psychiatric and social factors. The social factors in particular are extremely important with regard to the elderly, since it has been found that the unmarried, the childless, and those of a lower social class, are more likely to be admitted to geriatric care.

The results of community research are often studied in order that certain services should be provided for the community, since the health and the mental health in particular, of an ever ageing population, is one of the major problems facing our society today.

The third purpose of community studies is to see if the existing services might be utilised more efficiently and of acute moment is the interface between the health and social services, and many of the general practice surveys have concentrated on this aspect. Within the Glasgow area, researchers Powell[16] and Taylor[22] at the Kilsyth and Woodside Health Centres respectively, are investigating the possibility of identifying those elderly people who are at risk, by means of Health Visitor interviews.

More academic researchers are concerned with the changes in performance of psychological tests with age, but the practical applications of these studies are not difficult to envisage, the implications being that the individuals' functioning within their life situation might well be affected by fall-off in certain task performance.

Many other community researchers are concerned with the multi-factorial concept of vulnerability of the aged to physical and social risks. These researchers take heed of Durkheim's Anomic theory[2] of the breakdown of traditional, social restraints and shared values as being one cause of the increase in the mental instability in an elderly person. This can be seen to be almost more appropriate to the situation the elderly person finds himself in than in any other age group. Since 1954 there has been much research done in this field, but most surveys of the elderly at home have tended to deal with a specific aspect of geriatric medicine, such as the physical state, the mental state, or social conditions, and only in the exceptional study has the elderly person been examined as a whole. This we attempted to do in Glasgow by assessing in detail physical, mental, social and nutritional components of these elderly people's lives.

The Derivation of the Population[6]

Six medical practices were chosen at random from Executive Council's lists within a defined area of Glasgow, three each from the north-west and west areas. These two areas are well contrasted socially. The north-west district consists predominantly of the working class who live in council housing and/or in old Victorian late 19th century tenements in various states of dilapidation. Tenements such as these, pose many problems for the general community and especially for the elderly. These tenements consist of three or four storey buildings containing nine or more separate households. The typical old tenement flat consists of one room, one kitchen, with cold water only, and a w.c., which may be located outside the house but within the tenement building on a common landing or access corridor, which is known in Glasgow as a "close". The w.c. is usually shared by two or three other tenants (see Figure 1). Some are immaculately kept, but others are not kept at all. The unstable and feckless families often drift into these areas and live with the aged as their neighbours. Happily this is an area of redevelopment and many of the elderly have been rehoused in corporation tenements and council property.

In the west end area the houses of the middle and upper working classes may be found. Tenements abound in this area since this is the Glasgow habit, but here they are well kept and well-faced buildings with ornamental walls, and gardens. The council housing in this area is good and well looked after by responsible tenants.

By an age stratification procedure and random selection, from a possible population of 17,000 people of 65 years of age and over, 300 subjects were examined in detail.

Psychiatric assessment was made as indicated (Table 1) and every individual received various psychometric tests (Table 2) and scores were noted.

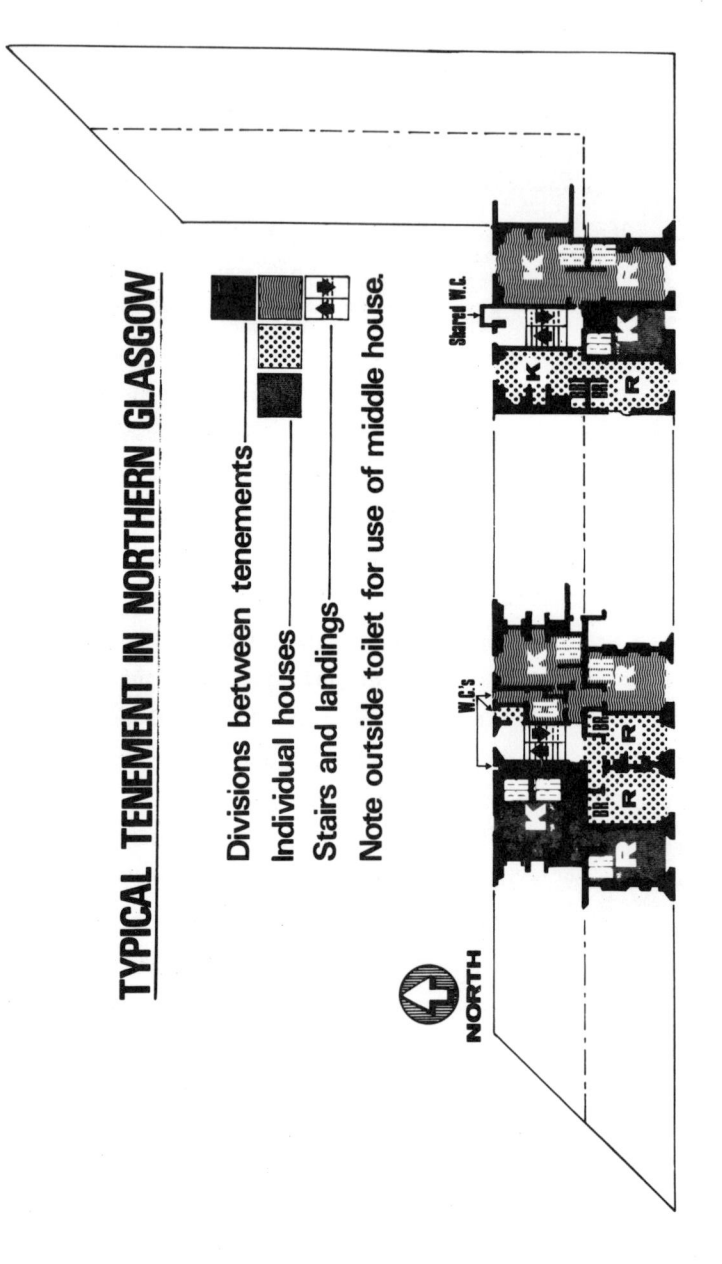

Figure 1

Table 1

PSYCHIATRIC SURVEY

Psychiatric Assessment was based on the following informational sources with regard to each person's diagnosis.

Source of Information	Location	Type of Information Obtained
General Practitioner	G.P.'s surgery	Medical, social, psychiatric background. family history.
G.P.'s medical records	G.P.'s surgery	Past history and work record.
Subject's family	Home	General medical history and background. Family inter-relationships.
Subject	Home/Clinic	As described elsewhere and including discussion of attitudes and sexual habits.
Test Battery	Home/Clinic	Psychometric Test Battery
Health Visitor	Home/Clinic	Social conditions, general background information.
Re-visit Survey	Home	Specific aims: symptoms enquired after, signs observed, any developments in subject's condition noted.
Further visits	Home	General psychiatric impression. Repetition of some psychometric tests, etc.

Table 2

PSYCHOMETRIC TEST BATTERY

(1) Crichton Vocabulary (abbreviated version)[19]

(2) The Coloured Progressive Matrices A, Ab and B[18]

(3) A Memory and Information Test (Appendix 2)

(4) The Crichton Behavioural Rating Scale[20]

(5) A short psychiatric Symptom Sign Inventory[5]

(6) A short Personality Inventory.[4]

It is amazing despite the diversions of purpose and the differences in methodology, and also cultural differences, that the prevalence rate with regard to organic psycho syndromes in Europe, show a remarkable degree of agreement. Table 3 shows the summary of surveys which have taken place since Sheldon's[21] famous study in 1948 with the percentage of dementia found in various countries. Some of these mental health surveys attempted also to divide dementia into severe and moderate/mild types. Table 4 is a diagrammatic representation of table 3 and shows the results of the attempts which have been made by the various authors to quantify the demented into mild/moderate or severe dementia categories. The proportional differences appearing here are considered to be due to the criteria used and it is interesting to note that in the two surveys by Scottish geriatricians, the more severe types of dementia form a very small proportion of the dementia rate as a whole.

One of the benefits of exploring different areas of research in a project such as this is the possibility of being able to correlate various findings.

These findings too can be used to define further populations.

For example, some 225 people in our study group of 300 appeared to be free of psychiatric abnormality. An important new population if one should wish to estimate normative data on the various psychometric tests involved in the test battery (Table 2).

Throughout the world, both physicians engaged in geriatric medicine, and psycho-geriatricians, have employed questionnaires termed and referred to by psychologists "Clinical Tests of the Sensorium", but which we refer to and understand in geriatrics as "Memory and Information Tests". There are a great many of these tests in common use today.

Table 3

PREVALENCE OF ORGANIC BRAIN SYNDROME
ACCORDING TO VARIOUS AUTHORS

Date	Author	Country	Dementia %	Severe	Mod./Mild
1948	Sheldon[21]	England	15·6	3·9	11·7
1951	Bremer[1]	Norway	not stated	2·5	–
1956	Essen-Moller[3]	Sweden	15·8	5·0	10·8
1962	Primrose[17]	Scotland	not stated	4·5	–
1964	Kay et al[13]	England	11·3	5·6	5·7
1964	Williamson et al[24]	Scotland	27·5	1·5	26
1965	Parsons[15]	Wales	14·4	4·4	10
1970	Hagnell[8]	Sweden	16·1	9·1	7·0
1972	Gilmore	Scotland	13·6	0·6	13·0

Table 4

Study	Total %	Inner value
GILMORE 1972	13.6%	.6
HAGNELL 1970[8]	16.1%	9.1
PARSONS 1965[15]	14.4%	4.4
WILLIAMSON 1964[24]	27.5%	1.5
KAY ET AL 1964[13]	11.3%	5.6
PRIMROSE 1962[17]	—	4.5
ESSEN-MOLLER 1956[3]	15.8%	5.0
BREMER 1951[1]	—	2.5
SHELDON 1948[21]	15.6%	3.9

% ORGANIC BRAIN SYNDROME ACCORDING TO VARIOUS AUTHORS

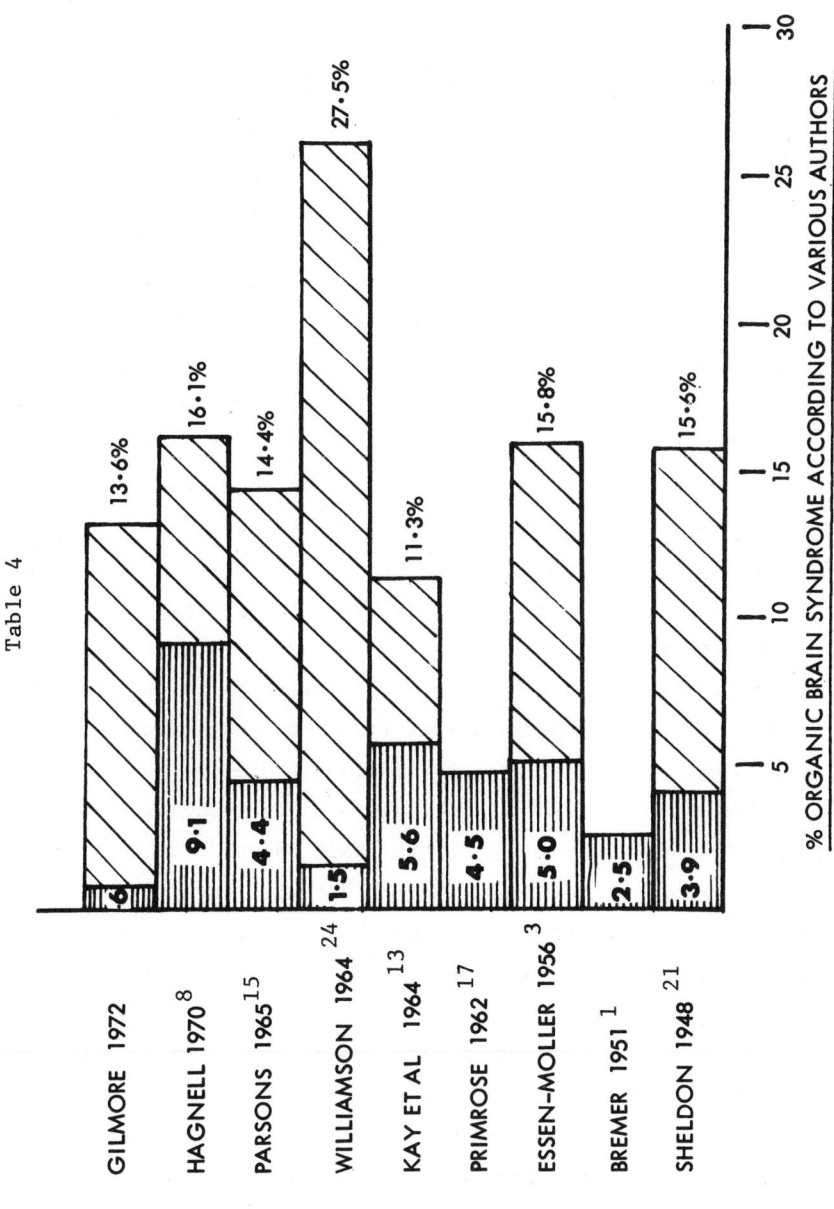

These inventories or questionnaires attempt to establish a diagnosis of and evaluate some of the patients' various cognitive functions. Table 5 shows the basic structure of these tests. Questions are directed to establishing the patients' appreciation of orientation, temporal, geographical, or personal, and appreciation of the interview situation. There is also always included a memory test for recent and remote events, with general information and knowledge. Testing of other abilities is sometimes included, for example, calculation and specific observations by an observer are sometimes also scored. We in Glasgow employed a similar 35-point scale test (appendix 1) to examine the distribution of scores by age, sex and diagnosis. Certainly, there appeared to be clear-cut differences in test scores between the "normals" and the demented people, as many other research workers have found also. Scores of 0-7 are obtained by the clinically severe demented; moderate between 7-17; and moderate/mild obtained scores of 17-27. What of the group, however, who scored between 27-35 on such a questionnaire, that all people in younger age groups, save mentally defective patients, score full points? It is hypothesised that this group may contain individuals who are beginning the dementing process.

The existence of such a category of individuals raises many questions. How often do definite brain symptoms develop later in these people? How long does the prodromal stage last, and how does it differ from the normal "senescent change"? Do such psychometric tests help to detect syndrome before it becomes clinically obvious?

Heron and Chown,[9] among many others, have stated and shown that the performance on some psychological tests tends to fall progressively at higher age groups. In their careful examination of age and function a battery of tests was given to normal people, who represented all ages from 20-28 years, and it was found that on Progressive Matrices the best score of the 70-79

Table 5

STRUCTURE OF MEMORY, INFORMATION AND ORIENTATION TESTS

1. <u>Orientation:</u> Temporal
   Geographical
   Personal
   Apprec. of Interview situation

2. <u>Memory:</u> Recent
   Remote

3. <u>General Information:</u> Current Affairs

4. <u>Other Intellectual Abilities:</u> Calculation
   Specific tests
   Specific observations

Appendix 1

Memory and Information Test

Preamble: I am going to give you a name and address. Later I will ask you to repeat them to me.

                William Morrison,
                7, Queen Street,
                Inverness.

Questions	Score

1. Serial 7's (100-93-86-79-72)
2. 1d. in 1/-
3. 3d. in 1/-
4. 3d. in 3/9
5. What day of the week is it today?
6. What day of the month is it?
7. What month is it?
8. What season is it?
9. What year is it?
10. What age are you? (allow 1 year error)
11. What year were you born?
12. In what month is your birthday?
13. What date is your birthday?
14. What is the name of this district?
15. What is the name of the next street?
16. Where did you see me last?
17. What sort of work do I do here?
18. What did you have for breakfast this morning?
19. Where were you born?
20. What school did you attend?
21. What was your teacher's name?
22. Who is on the British throne?
23. Who was on the throne before her?
24. What is the name of the present prime minister?
25. Who was the prime minister before him?
26. What were the dates (years) of the First World War? Start?   Finish?
27. What were the dates (years) of the Second World War? Start?   Finish?
28. How long have you been at your present address?
29. Can you remember the name and address I gave you at the beginning?
30. Can you remember my name?
31. Can you remember Sister's name?

Total Test Score: _____

35

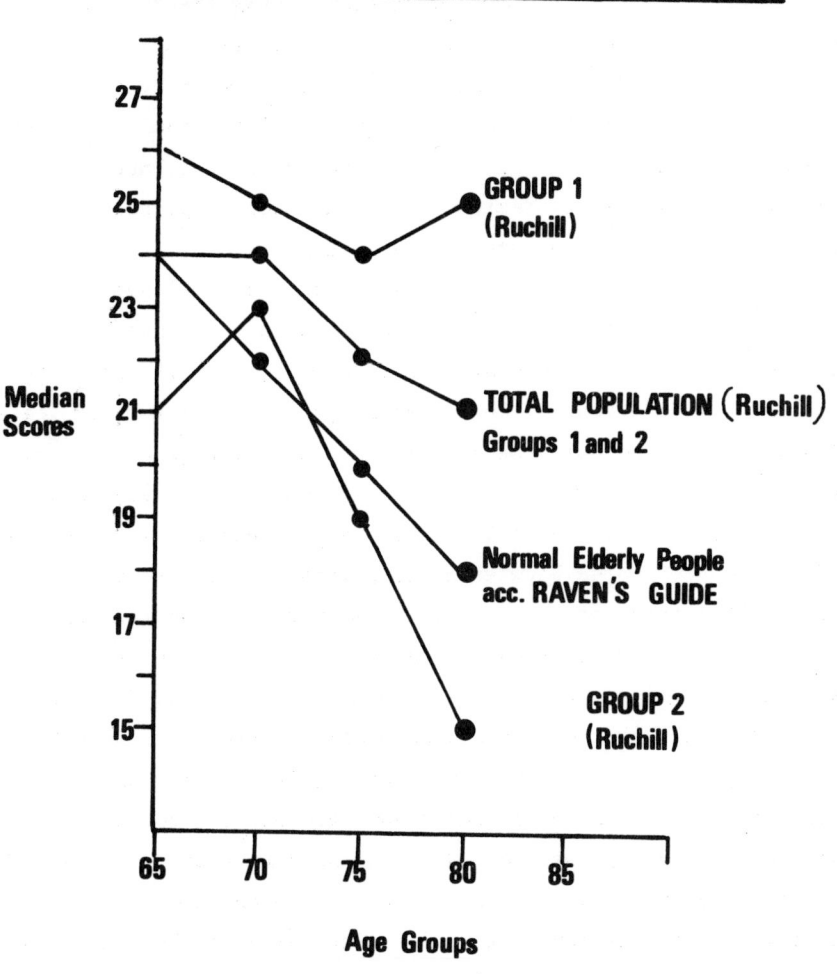

Figure 2

year old males was equal to the average score of the 20-29 year old group, and many of these older groups achieved very poor scores indeed.

Figure 2 shows some interesting points which can be gathered from the scores from our own population, using the Progressive Matrices.[18] Shown on this figure are the median exterpolated values, as quoted in the guide to progressive matrices. The authors of the manual state that their original population consists of normal healthy old people, and indeed this normative data is quoted in many textbooks, and has been duplicated by repeated use in many papers, by psychologists.

The fiftieth percentile scores of our 'normal' population, which consisted of 225 'normals', that is to say those people who appear to have no psychiatric abnormality at all, neither organic nor functional. The other lines on this figure indicate how these 225 'normals' behave on the progressive matrices[18] when they are arbitrarily divided by means of their scores on the Research Memory and Information Test (Appendix 1). A group of 113 people scored between 31-35 points whereas group 2 consisted of a group of 112 people who scored 27-31 on the Memory and Information Test, these therefore being the lower scorers. As can be seen group 1 appears to behave differently from group 2, although the combined population's behaviour resembles results given both in the manual for the Progressive Matrices[18] and those results of Heron and Chown[9] and other authors. Why should these groups separate so well and behave so uniquely differently on a selection procedure of siphoning off by a crude memory and information test, which clinically has been used for years to detect dementia? Is it perhaps that previous results of the psychologists have included within their population individuals who are already exhibiting pathological changes, as well as those who are undergoing normal senescent change. However, before one could come to any definite conclusions about such performance it would be necessary to remember that when one is studying the effects of increasing age on the behaviour and psychological functioning of individuals, the cross-sectional study is often an improper tool. In the cross-sectional study we often are only measuring an environmental effect compounded of an age effect and a cohort effect at one point in time.

There is very little information about the later history of these interesting groups of people who have lower scores on this type of test however. We are now following our original 300 over a period of three years, repeating all the original psychometric test battery and reinterviewing every subject and their relatives in their homes, establishing the cause of death if this has occurred, from both general practitioner and general records, and relating these data to our original findings.

If indeed it were to be found from this longitudinal study that this group with lower scores were more vulnerable to contract organic brain syndrome or intellectual deterioration, this would mean that such a simple test could be used to screen larger populations, with perhaps the possibility that these individuals might be investigated at an earlier stage in the onset of organic brain disorder. A more pragmatic view would be that these individuals might be buttressed or supported in some way within the community before the tidal wave of over-population hits the hospital services.

The mental health of the elderly in the community is worthy of much further study, but all students of different disciplines need to combine to examine the inter-relationship of men and women and health and in sickness, within and with regard to the community in which they have lived, worked, married, borne their children, and finally spent their old age, if preventative aspects of psychogeriatrics are to be investigated with any success.

References

1. Bremer, J. (1951). A social psychiatric investigation of a small community in N. Norway. Acta. Psych. Scand. Suppl. 62, English Ed.

2. Durheim (1952). Suicide: a study in sociology, London, Routledge and Kegan Paul.

3. Essen-Moller, E. (1956). Individual traits and morbidity in a Swedish rural population. Acta. Psych. Neurol. Scand. Suppl. 100.

4. Eysenck, H.J. (1959). Manual of the Maudsley Personality Inventory. London, University of London Press.

5. Foulds, G.A. and Hope, K. The Manual of the Symptom-Sign Inventory. University of London Press.

6. Gilmore, A.J.J. and Caird, F.I. (1972). Locating the elderly at home. Age and Ageing, $\underline{1}$, 30.

7. Grad, J. and Sainsbury, P. (1965). An evaluation of the effect of caring for the aged at home. Psychiatric Disorders in the Aged, Manchester. Geigy, 225 (U.K. Ltd.).

8. Hagnell, O. (1970). Disease expectancy and incidence of mental illness amongst the aged. Acta. Psych. Scand. Suppl. 219, 83.

9. Heron, A. and Chown, S. (1967). Age and Function. Pub. J.A. Churchill Ltd., London.

10. H.M.S.O. (1970). Services for the Elderly with Mental Disorders. Scottish Health Services Council.

11. Irving, G., Robinson, R.A. and McAdam, W. (1970). The validity of some cognitive tests in the diagnosis of dementia. Brit. J. Psych., $\underline{117}$, 149.

12. Isaacs, B. (1972). Survival of the Unfittest. Routledge and Kegan Paul.

13. Kay, D.W., Beamish, P. and Roth, M. (1964). Old age mental disorders. In: Newcastle-upon-Tyne, Part I, Study of Prevalence. Brit. J. Psych., $\underline{110}$, 146.

14. Neilsen, J. (1962). Geronto-psychiatric period-prevalence investigation in a geographically delimited population. Acta. Psych. Scand., $\underline{38}$, 307.

15 Parsons, P.L. (1965). Mental health of Swansey's old folk. J. Prev. Soc. Med., $\underline{19}$, 43.

16 Powell, C. and Crombie, A. Validation of health visitor questionnaire. Awaiting publication 1973.

17 Primrose, E.J.R. (1962). Psychiatric Illness – A Community Study, London. Tavistock Publications.

18 Raven, J.C. (1965). Guide to using the Coloured Progressive Matrices, London. H.K. Lewis & Co.

19 Raven, J.C. (1965). Guide to using the Coloured Progressive Matrices with Crichton Vocabulary Scale. H.K. Lewis & Co.

20 Robinson, R.A. (1965). Crichton Behavioural Rating Scale, p. 203. Psychiatric Disorders in the Elderly. Geigy (UK) Ltd., Manchester.

21 Sheldon (1948). Social Medicine of Old Age. Oxford University Press, London.

22 Taylor, B. Health Centres and the Elderly. Health Bulletin. 1973 in press.

23 Townsend, P. (1957). The Family Life of Old People. London. Routledge and Kegan, Paul.

24 Williamson, J. et al. (1964). Old people at home: their unreported needs. Lancet, $\underline{ii}$, 117.

ENVIRONMENT AND MENTAL HEALTH

THOMAS S. WILSON

Consultant Geriatrician
Barncoose Hospital, Redruth

My theme is environment and mental health. It may well be a reflection on the medical profession that, when a doctor is asked to talk about health, his immediate reaction is to think about ill-health; and to consider the factors involved in the production of this state of affairs. I hope you will forgive me if I take this approach, and deal briefly with the main elements in producing mental disturbance in old people. None of them may be considered in isolation. Like a jigsaw puzzle they fit together to produce the total picture of infirmity. Perhaps this may not be a wholly correct analogy, because some of the pieces may be variable, and alter the picture from time to time. The mental state is essentially a dynamic one, which is constantly changing in response to altered circumstances, rather than a fixed and immutable pattern. However, there are probably some pieces in this jigsaw puzzle which are permanently established and which determine the final outcome to a considerable extent.

What are the factors in each of us which influence how we shall grow old mentally - if we live long enough to do so?

1. GENETIC

It has been said that if we wish to grow old gracefully, we must choose our parents carefully. Insurance companies regard long-living parents as a good risk testimonial, and no doubt they have satisfactory statistical grounds for taking this view.

Personality types are also considered to be genetically determined, in the same way as red hair or a Roman nose may be passed from one generation to another. The type of personality may not determine whether or not we dement in old age, but it certainly has an affect on how we dement. Some of us may be acceptable as pleasantly "pixilated" old people, whilst others may become insufferably paranoid and unpleasant dements. Larsen and Sjogien[7] have postulated a specific gene which may be involved in those developing degenerative changes of brain cells.

2. AFFECTIVE DISORDERS

I do not propose, as a physician, to stray too far into the realms of psychiatry. The basic difference in approach of the two disciplines might be regarded as the emphasis on the brain on the one hand, and on the mind on the other. Perhaps even more in old people than in any other age group, the importance of the inter-play of organic and functional elements is evident. The multifactorial aspect of infirmity in senescence is just as true in the psychiatric disorders as it has been found to be in physical infirmities.

3. DEMENTIA

As one of the commonest psychiatric disorders of old age and probably that with the greatest impact, I would like to consider the problem of dementia.

Normal senescence involves an increasing rigidity and accentuation of patterns of behaviour which have been established in earlier life. Classically the miser is depicted as an old man, yet his penny pinching tendencies presumably, have always been a feature of his make-up, and have become more marked with the passage of years.

Luckily, not only our unpleasant characteristics are involved in the process. Some old people present with a serenity and tranquility which is a pleasure to behold. The borderline between normal and pathological ageing is ill-defined.

There are two main factors in the production of dementia:
(a) organic changes in the brain;
(b) the reaction of the individual personality to these changes and to physical and environmental stress.

(a) <u>Organic Changes in the Brain</u>

These may be classified on a histological basis into three main groups: primarily neuropathic, primarily arteriopathic, and a group in which both these factors are operative. The "chronic brain syndrome" is the result of the loss of irreplaceable brain cells, either by a degenerative process of the neurones, by cerebral infarction resulting from ischaemia, or less commonly by cell death due to other reasons. The clinical differentiation into the two main groups of senile and arteriosclerotic dementia is not always easy. Based mainly on the mode of onset, and the presence or absence of focal neurological signs, it is frequently proved to be inaccurate on subsequent post-mortem. Yet the differentiation has more than academic value. A number of workers have shown that the natural history of the conditions are different, and that the expectation of life is significantly less in senile dementia than in the arteriopathic type.

(b) <u>Personality</u>

Although the organic changes in the brain determine the efficiency of this organ, the reaction of the personality of the individuals is equally relevant to the mode of presentation of his disability.

How does one define personality? The definitions in the literature are for the most part self-defeating in that they are so comprehensive as to be quite incomprehensible - for example "the integrated organisation of all cognitive, affective, conative and physical characteristics of an individual as it manifests itself in focal distinctions from others".[13] I prefer the simplest, which defines an individual's personality as "his unique pattern of traits".[6]

We have noted the hereditary factors involved in personality. However, up-bringing, early background and environmental stress all play an important part in developing this pattern. It is interesting to reflect that the dementias which we see today are occurring in patients whose personality traits were established around the turn of the century. One wonders how the present tempo of living, the so-called permissive society, and other traumata of the current social scene will affect the presentation of the dementias of the future. The mature personality has been defined by Allport[2] as having:

(i) an extended and creative outlook;
(ii) insight into his own motives and abilities with a sense of humour;
(iii) a unifying philosophy of life.

In contrast, the personality which is liable to breakdown is one where the individual is "rigid" in his attitude towards himself and others, without insight into his failings, dogmatic, obstinate and intolerant.

Such traits are obviously a handicap at any age, but when confronted with the stresses of ageing, they may give rise to unbalanced reactions.

Perhaps most significant with regard to previous personality in the production of senile psychosis is a consideration of basic histo-pathology. One is often disappointed in finding little relevent correlation between the clinical findings and the degree of cerebral pathology.

I adhere to Gitelson's view[4] when he said that:

"Elderly people with more or less well-balanced personalities are able to cope with a considerable amount of cerebral damage, while less well-balanced personalities may produce a frank psychosis with a minimum of cerebral pathology."

4. ENVIRONMENTAL STRESS

It has been suggested that environmental stress, even in adult life, may accelerate the ageing process. Subjective observations by Bergman[3] indicated that Australian survivors from Japanese P.O.W. camps frequently appeared older than their years would suggest, and Professor Roth[12] has raised the query whether prolonged emotional disturbance produces adrenal overactivity, and whether this may affect ageing.

I think that everyone would agree that environmental stress occurring in old age is an important factor in the production of psychiatric disturbance.

The insults of ageing include the decline in physical and intellectual potential with the passage of time. This is not peculiar to advanced years, however. The Olympic swimmer is past his prime when he leaves his teens, and the international rugby player tends to be dropped when he is past 30!

The traditional milestones in old age which have to be passed successively are retirement and bereavement. To this I would add a third - rejection.

(a) Retirement

Affleck[1] has described this as:

"The antithesis of graduation, and often amounts to a public disrobing ceremony in which the victim faces the prospect of reduced income, no occupation, and ex-communication from the company of his business friends".

I wonder if this is really the bogey it has been made out to be? I think that the individual who finds retirement an obstacle is one whose resources are already strained to the limit. To many it is an opportunity to a fuller life, rather than an invitation to a wake. I think that those who fall at this hurdle would not have successfully completed many more laps in an event.

There is little real evidence that retirement plays a significant part in the production of mental illness in old age. Indeed, as Jacqueline Grad[5] has pointed out, most of the evidence suggests the contrary. In particular, the fact that women, who are rarely affected by retirement, are no less likely to become mentally ill in the retirement period than men are, although depressive illness has a somewhat greater frequency in females than in males. One of the few positive reports to support the view of an adverse influence of retirement is that of Logan and Cushion,[8] who found in their report on morbidity in general practice a higher rate of patients consulting for depression among retired than among working men over 65.

There has been a vogue for pre-retirement clinics, designed to prepare people for a fruitful retirement. I think it is fair to say that these have not been an unqualified success. Perhaps this is because the people who take the trouble to attend them are those who are not really in need of their facilities. Those who do rarely appear.

(b) Bereavement

It has been shown that bereavement has a significant mortality rate. Parkes et al. in 1969[11] in a follow-up study of over 4,000 males of over 54 years, whose wives had died in 1957 showed an increase in mortality in the first 4 years following bereavement than would be expected on the basis of data relating to married men of the same age. The increase was particularly marked during the first 6 months following bereavement when it amounted to more than 40%.

Other studies have similarly indicated an increased mortality following bereavement, and MacMahon and Pugh[9] showed that loss of a spouse pre-disposes to suicide in the period immediately following. They estimated that the suicide risk is maximal in the year following loss, when it is about 2½ times greater than four or more years later.

(c) Isolation

Other reasons for social isolation have been the subject of numerous studies. These have examined two main groups of social deprivation - lack of material things, as measured by social class, income and housing, etc., and lack of friends or family, as measured by marital state, household composition, number of contacts and so on. The results have been rather equivocal. As Jacqueline Grad[5] points out, they all fail to show any positive evidence for a relationship between social class and poverty, and mental illness in old age, but they all find some evidence that the type of social interaction people have is so related. There is clearly some relationship between the amount of company a person keeps and his tendency to become mentally ill in old age.

(d) Rejection

All those who work with old people will be familiar with what might be called "the rejection syndrome", which probably produces a mortality as great as, if not greater, than that of bereavement. The behaviour disorders of psychiatric illness are more prone to produce rejection by relatives than even severe physical infirmities. A vicious circle is thus established, where further deterioration in mental physical status results.

One is often confronted by this dilemma in geriatric wards, where the relatives are unwilling to accept the patient back in view of previous experience, yet to acquaint the patient of this fact will inevitably result in a deterioration in morale and physical well-being with a not insignificant increase in mortality.

Perhaps the best solution to this problem is to break this vicious circle before it becomes rigidly established. Adequate and early relief to the strained household is important, by domiciliary support, day hospital, or by intermittent admission. The level of tolerance of a family is considerably raised by the knowledge that the social and hospital services are available to fall back upon when the crisis arises.

5. <u>RAPIDITY OF CHANGE</u>

We have discussed the physical and environmental factors in the production of psychiatric disorders. Quantitatively they are important. The extent of organic brain damage is relevant, as is the degree of environmental stress. Equally important, however, is the mode of onset of these insults. The human organism requires time to adapt to change, and this is particularly the case in senescence, when mechanisms of adaptation are less efficient. Organic change and environmental stress, even of severe degree, is much better tolerated and produces less impact, if it has been slow in onset, whereas lesser degrees which have occurred suddenly tend to produce much more florid results.

<u>SHELTERED ENVIRONMENT</u>

Finally, I would like to comment on the facilities available for old people with mental infirmity.

The aim of psycho-geriatric services is to provide adequate assessment of the factors involved in the disability, appropriate treatment, both physical and psychiatric, on discharge to the most suitable environment. This may mean a return to the community, resettlement in a residential home, or in a long-stay hospital, either geriatric or psychiatric.

Many local authorities provide special residential homes for old people with mental infirmity, in addition to the more usual homes for the physically frail. A desirability of such homes has

recently been queried by Meacher,[10] following a sociological study. He has raised objections to what he calls "separatist homes" on the grounds of:
  (i) fewer such homes, therefore more geographically scattered, and residents receive vastly fewer visits;
  (ii) he considered they encouraged greater segregation of residents;
  (iii) he criticised what he calls the psychological implications of separation.

He advocated the dispersal of mentally infirm residents on an equal basis with rational residents in all homes.

His opinions are completely contrary to our experience of special residential homes in Cornwall, and do not in my view, stand up to detailed scrutiny.

It would be unfortunate if this report should inhibit in any way the further development of special residential homes, which have a considerable role in the future care of old people with irreversible mental disturbance.

The planning of such homes is important. The size is considered to be of considerable relevance. Few self-respecting local authorities would now contemplate building a home for more than 50 to 60 residents. Indeed, I am given to understand that the Department would be unwilling to give loan sanction for the erection of any home with more than 50 places. Any larger, and there is a danger of it developing an "institutional atmosphere". I think this is a valid concept, and that there is an optimum size of a group of people who can live together beyond which the individual tends to lose his sense of personal identity - a condition which used to be manifest in the large institutions by the development of institutional apathy. There are parallels to this in other species, for example, the rigid hierarchy of the "pecking order" suddenly breaks down in a group of chickens when the group is enlarged beyond a certain degree, another example of loss of personal identity.

Given that this is the case with regard to the size of welfare homes, it has always seemed illogical to me that similar considerations have not been applied in the planning for long-stay geriatric patients. These differ from residents in welfare homes only in the extent of their disabilities and the degree of care and attention they require from the staff. I can see no reason whatever why the environment in which they live should differ substantially from that of residents in welfare homes. This is a subject to which the hospital planners and sociologists should give considerably more thought.

I wholeheartedly agree with Professor Ferguson Anderson on the point which he made at this meeting about the appropriate size of hospitals for continued care. His is the first voice of authority which I have heard raise this important consideration. Such hospitals are essentially a substitute for the patient's own home, and the environment of care they provide should have a domestic rather than a hospital orientation.

In order to decide the appropriate environment for someone who needs continued sheltered care an effective system of assessment is required - the Psycho-Geriatric Assessment Unit. This is a joint responsibility of psychiatrist and geriatrician where the benefits of both disciplines can be brought to bear on the problems of each individual patient.

References

1. Affleck, J.W. (1949). Personality factors in the senile psychoses. Paper read to the Medical Society for the Care of the Elderly. Liverpool Meeting.

2. Allport, G.W. (1937). Personality : A psychological interpretation. New York. Holt.

3. Bergman, R.A.M. (1948). Who is Old? Death rate in Japanese concentration camps as criterion of age. J. Geront., 3, 14.

4. Gitelson, M. (1948). Emotional problems of elderly people. Geriatrics, III, 135.

5. Grad, J. (1971). Recent developments in psycho-geriatrics. A symposium. British Journal of Psychiatry. Special Publication No. 6.

6. Guilford, J.P. (1959). Personality. McGraw Hill Series in psychology. McGraw Hill Book Co. New York, Toronto and London.

7. Larson, T., Sjogien, T. and Jacobson, G. (1963). Senile dementia. Acta Psychiatrica Scandanavia. 39 Suppl. 167.

8. Logan, W.P.D. and Cushion, A.A. (1960). Morbidity statistics from general practice. General Register Office Studies in Medical Population Subjects. Vol. II, No. 14. London, H.M.S.O.

9. McMahon, B. and Pugh, T.F. (1965). Suicide in the widowed. American Journal of Epidemiology., 81, 23.

10. Meacher, M. (1972). Taken for a ride : special residential homes for the elderly mentally infirm : a study of separation in social policy. Community Medicine, No. 3325. Vol. 128, No. 1.

11. Parkes, C.M., Benjamin, B. and Fitzgerald, R.G. (1969). Broken heart : a statistical study of increased mortality among widowers. Brit. Med. J., I, 740.

12. Roth, M. (1965). Psychiatric aspects of old age in relation to the problem of ageing. Symposium of World Psychiatric Association.

13. Warren, H.C. (1934). Dictionary of psychology. Boston Houghton Mifflia.

DRUGS AND MEMORY

THOMAS G. JUDGE

Consultant Physician in Geriatric Medicine
Stobhill Hospital, Glasgow

Until quite recently it has been believed that all age changes in mental function are in the direction of decline, that is to say, loss of concentration, loss of memory, loss of cognition (Figure 1), and as Wechsler[9] noted, many influences are operative (Table 1). It may be that these are not simply the changes of age but disease changes brought about by disease processes, but this fine distinction is more a matter of philosophical debate than practical concern. The picture is complicated in many old people by the high instance of depression to which Dr. Anne Gilmore has referred earlier, producing a further apparent decline in cognition and function.

The end product of mental impairment in the elderly is referred to as dementia which literally means loss of mind, but has come to mean irreversible loss of mind. We all recognise the principal varieties of dementia; arteriosclerotic dementia which is characterised by its intermittency and "senile" dementia characterised by its irrevocable progressiveness. Since dementia is probably an incorrect name and since patients

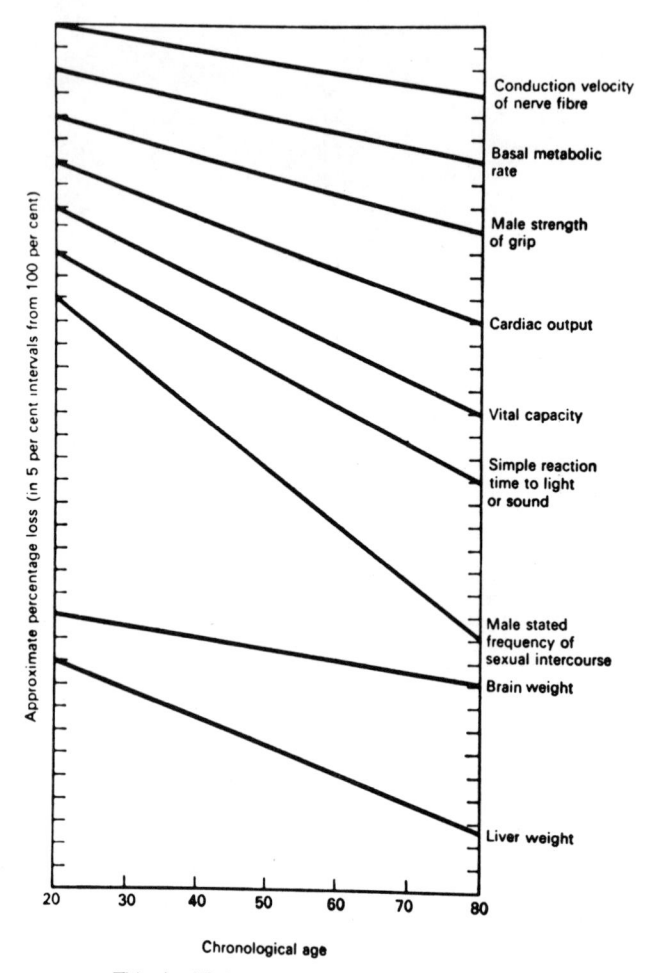

This simplified diagram illustrates relative age differences for several biological variables expressed as a percentage loss of function from the age of 20.

Figure 1

This figure is reproduced by kind permission of the author D.B. Bromley, and the Publishers Penguin Books from the Psychology of Human Ageing.

Table 1

Adult Intelligence

Test	Method	Age Effect	Pertinant Influences
Verbal Attainments	Vocabulary Information Comprehension	+-	Attainments not capacity Speed unimportant Immediate memory unimportant
Short-term memory	Digit Span Forwards and Backwards	+	Very short-term retention Speed unimportant Simple task
Mental Arithmetic	Simple calculations	++	Well practised skill Little reasoning Simple task
Rational thinking	Raven's Matrices Similarities	+++	Abstract thought Logical thought Principle selection Speed Capacity
Mental Speed	Digit symbol Substitution	+++	Complex procedure Speed Capacity
Non-Verbal Intelligence	Picture arrangement Picture completion Block design Object assembly	++++	Short-term memory Logical thought Abstract thought Speed Attention Capacity

This table is reproduced by the kind permission of the author and publishers from "The Measurement and appraisal of Adult Intelligence", by D. Wechsler. Published by Bailliere and Tindall, London, 1959.

with arteriosclerotic dementia frequently do not have arteriosclerosis and since we are all committed to the abolition of senility these names are rather like the Lord Privy Seal who is neither a Lord nor a Privy nor a seal. The term brain failure is to be preferred and can usually be subdivided into acute and chronic.[4] Table 2 shows the principle causes of brain failure in the elderly. This change of name helps to create an environment in which treatment is possibly in contrast to the therapeutic nihilism of the older nomenclature. Treatable conditions which lead to brain failure must be dealt with before attempting to use non-specific drugs which improve mental function. Recently an increased number of drugs have appeared on the British market reputed to improve mental function in the elderly in diverse pharmacological ways. I have called these drugs psycho-anabatic* agents because of their non-specific action and common end result. When these drugs were first introduced they were often claimed to be cerebral vasodilators. We know that the cerebral vessels can dilate, for example, carbon dioxide[2] is a very potent cerebral vasodilator but whether or not such cerebral vasodilators improve brain function is open to serious doubt. The measurement of cerebral blood flow is very difficult in the elderly, indeed in any patient, since internal carotid and internal jugular canilation are unacceptable ethically in human beings. The inhalation Xenon techniques are a possibility, but at the moment there is serious doubt about their validity[5] and even more there is a serious lack of correlation between blood flow studies and mental testing function.[1] My view is that in the present state of knowledge it is more practical to measure the function end point, that is to say, to take elderly patient, see whether under rigorously controlled conditions the measurable components of mental function can be improved with these drugs.[6]

---

*From the Greek ana to move and batic - upwards.

Table 2

Some Causes of Brain Failure in Old Age

1. Structural damage to the brain:

    e.g. cerebral infarction, cerebral haemorrhage, cerebral tumour (primary or secondary), 'senile dementia', subdural haematoma.

2. Disorders of the cerebral circulation:

    e.g. carotid insufficiency, systemic hypotension, congestive cardiac failure.

3. Metabolic brain disorders:

    e.g. hypoxia, uraemia, dehydration, electrolyte disorder, thyroid disease, hypoglycaemia, vitamin deficiency (of vitamin B_{12} or folate).

4. Epilepsy.

5. Drug toxicity:

    e.g. poisoning with barbiturate, phenothiazines, alcohol, digitalis, etc.

This table is reproduced by permission of the authors and publishers from "The Assessment of the Elderly Patient" by F.I. Caird and T.G. Judge. Pitman Medical, London, 1973.

In my own early work I was concerned with the correct placing of patient, that is to say, whether these drugs can influence incontinence and activities of daily living, and the Longmore Score (Figure 2) developed by MacLeod and myself in Edinburgh, was our first attempt to study this.[6] Using this group of tests I was unable to demonstrate any drug action from Cosaldon (Hexyl Theobromine and Nicotinic Acid), Lucidril (Meclofenoxate), or Hexopal (Inositol nicotinate). This of course does not rule out drug action with these substances; these tests may have been inappropriate but certainly no powerful action was present in these patients. In a more recent study using sophisticated tests, Cyclospasmol (Cyclandelate) was shown to be effective in healthy elderly volunteers in the community.[7] Praxilene (Naftidrofuryl) in a recent study in severely impaired hospital in-patients produced significant improvement in some.[8] All these studies were carried out with patients in a steady state using double blind technique with crossover.

At the moment I think it is fair to say that we must no longer regard dementia as the burned-out end product of disease for which there is no treatment, but as a dynamic state requiring urgent research. Over the next few years numerous new drugs will appear for the treatment of brain failure in the elderly and we must be highly critical of them and assess them carefully least we waste our resources, or even worse, fail to treat a treatable condition when highly potent drugs become available.

The Longmore Disability Score

Assessment of mental function and daily activities

I am now going to tell you a name and address and the names of two flowers and their colours and I will ask you later to repeat them back.

>James Anderson,
>9 King's Road, Perth:
>
>red tulip; white daisy

Intelligence

Now I am going to ask you a number of short questions which I ask everyone:

		Score
1.	Serial 7's (100 - 93 - 86 - 79)?	0 to 2
2.	How many 1d. are there in a 1/-d?	0 to 2
3.	How many 3d. are there in 3/9d?	0 to 2
4.	What day of the week is it?	0 to 2
5.	What month is it?	0 to 2
6.	What year is it?	0 to 2
7.	What year were you born?	0 to 2
8.	What is the name of this place?	0 to 2
9.	What sort of place is it?	0 to 2
10.	What sort of work do I do here?	0 to 2
11.	What school did you attend?	0 to 2
12.	Do you remember any of your teachers' names?	0 to 2
13.	Who is on the British throne?	0 to 2
14.	Who was on the throne before her?	0 to 2
15.	What is the name of the present Prime Minister?	0 to 2
16.	Who was the Prime Minister before him?	0 to 2
17.	What were the dates (years) of the First World War - start and finish?	0 to 2
18.	What were the dates (years) of the Second World War - start and finish?	0 to 2
19.	What is my name?	0 to 2
20.	What is Sister's name?	0 to 2

Recall

21.	Can you remember the name and address and the flowers and their colours which I gave you?	up to 10

Daily Activities

	Score
Toilet:	
Needs help in toilet	2
Uses bedpan or commode	5
Occasionally incontinent	10
Persistently incontinent	15
Doubly incontinent	20
Dressing:	
Needs a little help	2
Needs much help	4
Cannot dress	5
Feeding:	
Needs to be fed	5
Mobility:	
Requires walking aid	3
Requires help of one	6
Requires help of two	10
Chairfast	15
Bedfast	20

Figure 2 (contd.)

References

1. Ball, J.A.C. and Taylor, A.R. (1967). Effect of Cyclandelate on mental function and cerebral blood flow in elderly patients. Brit. Med. J., $\underline{3}$, 525.

2. Bernsmeier, A., Gottstein, U., Held, K. and Nedermayer, W. (1967). The stroke - pathogenesis, course and prognosis. In: Annals of Life Insurance Medicine, Springer, Berlin.

3. Bromley, D.B. (1966). The Psychology of Human Ageing. Penguin Books, Middlesex.

4. Caird, F.I. and Judge, T.G. (1973). The Assessment of the Elderly Patient. Pitman Medical, London.

5. Corbett, J.L., Eidleman, B.H. and Debarge, O. (1972). Modification of cerebralvaso constriction with hypoventilation in normal man by thymoxamine. Lancet, $\underline{2}$, 461.

6. Judge, T.F. (1971). The Assessment of the Older Patient. "Assessment in Cerebrovascular Insufficiency" Ed. Stocke, G., Kuhn, R.A., Hall, P., Becker, G. and Van der Veen, E., Springer, Stugart.

7. Judge, T.G. et al. (1973). Cyclandelate and mental functions: a double blind cross-over trial in normal elderly subjects. Age and Ageing, $\underline{2}$, 121.

8. Judge, T.G. and Urquhart, Anne (1972). Naftidofuryl - a double blind cross-over study in the elderly. Current Medical Research and Opinion, $\underline{1}$, No. 3.

9. Wechsler, D. (1958). The Measurement and Appraisal of Adult Intelligence. 4th Ed. Bailliere, Tindal and Cox, London.

ADVANCES IN TECHNIQUES OF DIAGNOSIS,
TREATMENT AND RESEARCH

RESEARCH IN GERIATRIC MEDICINE

Chairman's Remarks

FRANCIS I. CAIRD

Senior Lecturer in Geriatric Medicine
University of Glasgow

Few would doubt the pressing need for research into the numerous medical problems of the elderly, but there are some who feel that the task of geriatrics and of those who practice it is solely to care for patients, and not to indulge in the pastime of research. This view is certainly erroneous, and is indeed arguably pernicious, because if one thing is certain, it is that if those who practice geriatrics do not themselves actively pursue research into the disorders of old age, no one else will. Conversely, there are many conditions, particularly for instance athero-sclerosis and chronic bronchitis, which are very common and important in old age, and yet are, in my own opinion, inappropriate topics for research by geriatricians, since these conditions clearly have their origins in middle age and should therefore be rightly regarded as in the province of those interested in the disorders of middle age.

Most of the important areas of geriatric research are represented in papers presented at this meeting. Simple clinical research must continue, both in the physical and psychiatric fields. Perhaps the most striking single recent example of the value of investigations of this kind is given by the work of Hurwitz and Adams on the problems of patients with stroke, and their recognition and management.[5] This constitutes a major advance in its own right, and is also perhaps the most important contribution of British geriatrics to the mainstream of clinical medicine. Also of great importance, for the next decade or so, will be continuance of the old-fashioned activity of clinico-pathological correlation. There is no doubt that much remains to be discovered, if not new diseases, at least new forms taken by old diseases in old age. Physicians in geriatric medicine, with continuing-care wards under their charge, have an unrivalled opportunity for the careful clinical investigation of elderly patients, to be followed in due course by appropriate and detailed pathological study. The correlation demonstrated between the pathological and clinical manifestations of senile dementia is an outstanding example of the proper use of these opportunities.[12]

Physiological studies seem more up-to-date. We need much more information about the disorders of physiological function shown by the elderly. Thus the elucidation of the abnormalities of temperature regulation in elderly patients who have recovered from hypothermia has made it clear that such abnormalities are not characteristic of all old people, but only of a few.[9] They indicate the need for thought about the management of such patients in the acute stage of their illness and after recovery, in order to prevent recurrence, and also about the very difficult problem of their detection, before the development of hypothermia. Closely linked with investigations of this kind, and perhaps of even greater immediate importance, are studies of the clinical pharmacology of old age. Unwanted reactions to many drugs increase in frequency with age, and the metabolism and thus the effects of drugs are clearly altered by common physiological changes in old age, of which the most clearly demonstrated to date are the consequences of reduction in glomerular filtration.

In an allied field are the nutritional disorders, which are now, at least in developed societies, almost confined to the elderly. Here much further work is necessary, especially perhaps on the identification of subclinical deficiencies of vitamins C and D,[10] and on the part played by the latter in the development of bone rarefaction in old age.[2,4,8,11] The demonstration of the frequency of potassium depletion[7] in the elderly constitutes a further challenge, in terms of its recognition and of the elucidation of its mechanism and consequences.

Doctors must never neglect the study of the social problems of old age, if only because so many of these have a very large underlying medical basis. Thus a recent social survey of disablement[3] goes into great detail about the causes of disability but does not attempt to establish these causes by clinical examination. When this is done, at least for the elderly living at home[1], the causes of disability are found to be very different from those confidently and authoritatively determined by non-medical means. Finally, operational research is of crucial importance both for proper planning for the future and for the evaluation of the efficacy of the various administrative defices to which geriatricians are perforce addicted. Thus for instance, despite the enthusiasm with which day hospitals are advocated, there is very little fact on which to base a rational view of the way in which they function and the benefits they confer.

These are some examples of the forms which research in geriatric medicine should take, and so enable a better understanding of the problems which the elderly encounter and for which they need help.

References

1. Akhtar, A.J., Broe, G.A., Crombie, A., McLean, W.M.R., Andrews, G.R. and Caird, F.I. (1973). Disability and dependence in the elderly at home. Age and Ageing, 2, 102.

2. Exton-Smith, A.N., Hodkinson, H.M. and Stanton, B.R. (1966). Nutrition and metabolic bone disease in old age. Lancet, ii, 999.

3. Harris, A.I. (1971). Handicapped and impaired in Great Britain. London, H.M.S.O.

4. Hodkinson, H.M. (1971). Fracture of the femur as a presentation of osteomalacia. Geront. Clin., 13, 189.

5. Hurwitz, L.J. and Adams, G.F. (1972). Rehabilitation of hemiplegia: indices of assessment and prognosis. Brit. med. J., 1, 94.

6. Hurwitz, N. and Wade, O.L. (1969). Intensive hospital monitoring of adverse reactions to drugs. Brit. med. J., i, 531.

7. Judge, T.G. (1972). Potassium metabolism in the elderly: In: Nutrition in Old Age, ed. Carlson, L.A. Almquist and Wiksell, Stockholm.

8. McLennan, W.J., Caird, F.I. and Macleod, C.C. (1972). Diet and bone rarefaction in old age. Age and Ageing, 1, 131.

9. McMillan, A.L., Corbett, J.L., Johnson, R.H., Smith, A.C., Spalding, J.M.K. and Wollner, L. (1967). Temperature regulation in survivors of accidental hypothermia of the elderly. Lancet, ii, 165.

10. Milne, J.S., Lonergan, M.E., Williamson, J., Moore, F.M.L., McMaster, R. and Percy, N. (1971). Leucocyte ascorbic acid levels and vitamin C intake in older people. Brit. med. J., iv, 383.

11. Nordin, B.E.C. (1971). Clinical significance and pathogenesis of osteoporosis. Brit. med. J., i, 571.

12. Tomlinson, B.E., Blessed, G. and Roth, M. (1970). Observations on the brains of demented old people. J. Neurol. Sci., 11, 205.

RECENT ADVANCES IN INCONTINENCE

PROFESSOR JOHN C. BROCKLEHURST

Professor of Geriatric Medicine
University of Manchester

In the last few years there has been no new major study related to incontinence either in the bladder or in the bowel. There have, however, been a number of additions to previous knowledge which are important and interesting, and these will be considered first in relation to urinary incontinence and secondly in relation to faecal incontinence.

Urinary Incontinence
Epidemiology

Incontinence is one aspect of dysuria of elderly people and aetologically the two are closely associated. Two recent surveys have added to and partly confirmed previous findings in elderly people in the community. These are those of Milne and his colleagues[16] who studied a representative population of people aged 62 and upwards in Edinburgh, and that of Brocklehurst and his colleagues[8] who studied a group of women aged 45 to 64 on the list of a general practice and compared these with findings previously obtained in women aged 65 and over from the same practice. While comparison between surveys of this type is often difficult because the questions asked are not exactly comparable, nevertheless, the survey which Milne and his colleagues carried out tends to confirm the incidence of dysuria found in previous studies by Sourander[20] and Brocklehurst et al.[7] The findings of the Edinburgh study are shown in Table 1.

No statistical association was found between incontinence and the presence of bacteriuria. An association between chronic brain syndrome and incontinence is found which is in keeping with findings previously reported by Isaacs and Walkey[12] and Brocklehurst.[2] The second study in which Brocklehurst and his colleagues compare findings of symptoms of dysuria in women above and below the age of 65 showed an exact similarity in the incidence of scalding and of precipitancy but nocturnal frequency was twice as common in women aged 65 and over as in the younger group and significant bacteriuria was 3% in the younger group compared to 20% in the older group. The younger group were not asked specifically about the incidence of incontinence but they were asked about stress incontinence of which 57% reported some stress incontinence present. This incidence of stress incontinence is similar to those reported by Namir and Middleton[17] and Wollin[23] among large numbers of younger women.

It seems to be well established now that nocturnal frequency of micturition in females is generally associated with loss of cortical inhibition over the sacral bladder centre. Evidence for this is, in the first place, that the degree of nocturnal frequency increases with age, that it is related to toy test performance, and that it is improved by anticholinergic drugs. This may not be the whole cause; the fact that old people may sleep less well and therefore waken more frequently during the night may contribute; again there may be some alteration in nyctohemeral excretion of urine, possibly associated with slight change in renal function. However, no evidence has been produced to support either of these theories.[2]

Table 1

(all figures %)

	Day Time Frequency	Nocturnal Frequency	Incontinence	Severe Incontinence
Males	33	49	25	5
Females	23	67	42	4.5

It is not intended to review the neurogenic basis of urinary incontinence in old age since this has been described on a number of previous occasions.[5] However, other possible causes of incontinence should be considered and other contributory factors.

One last word on the incidence of incontinence might be devoted to the surveys of Isaacs and his colleagues[13] who, comparing admissions to a medical and a geriatric ward, showed that incontinence as a presenting symptom was present in 8% of patients admitted to the medical ward and 51% of those admitted to the geriatric ward. Also that 40% of old people dying at home were incontinent. These are simply measures of the burden placed on relatives and on nurses in geriatric departments by this continuing problem of urinary incontinence.

Anatomy

It would seem that continence in the human is assured partly by the low resting pressure of the urine in the bladder and partly by the physical properties of the urethra and the effect of its surrounding elastic tissue. The external sphincter itself is not necessarily for the maintenance of continence, although by its voluntary contraction it is able to stop micturition. The internal sphincter is not an anatomical reality and, in fact, the disposition of muscle fibres round the bladder outlet shows that their contraction is likely to open the outlet rather than to close it (see Woodburne).[24]

Another interesting feature of the ageing urinary tract is the presence of a degree of prolapse of the urethral mucosa in a large number of elderly women. This was investigated by S.M. Dymock (unpublished) who examined 100 consecutive female geriatric patients and found such a prolapse in 69 of them. In nine of these there was a caruncle; in the remainder there were varying degrees of prolapse. There was an association with decensus in as much as all patients who showed prolapse of the bladder or rectum also showed prolapse of the urethral mucosa but this accounted only for 9 of the 69 patients with this urethrocele. Dymock found a significant correlation between the urethrocele and incontinence. The significance of this finding is not at present known.

Histology

Histological change in the ageing bladder has been related partly to the fact that oestrogens seem to affect the epithelium of parts of the bladder and urethra in the female just as they affect the epithelium of the genital tract, and Judge has shown that the use of oestrogens has some apparent affect in incontinence in elderly people.[15] Also the fact that many urologists practice resection of the neck of the bladder (a procedure which is not without danger) in elderly women who have symptoms of dysuria associated with a significant amount of residual urine. The reason for this so called bladder neck stenosis is not known. Brocklehurst[4] carried out a limited histological study of the bladder outlet in bladders obtained from aged women dying in hospital and showed that the histological changes were entirely non-specific - those of oedema, round cell infiltration and fibrosis. There was no evidence of hypertrophy of any analogue of the female prostate (e.g. the para-urethral glands). The finding of stratified squamous epithelium in the place of transitional epithelium[19] indicates a possible reason why oestrogens should be effective in dysuria and suggests that some forms of dysuria (e.g. urethral syndrome) may be associated with oestrogen based changes in the menstrual cycle.

Treatment of Incontinence

The use of Faradism and pelvic floor exercises in stress incontinence has been described by Tanner[22] and this form of treatment now seems well established as a first approach to stress incontinence, which is not associated with severe desencus of the pelvic organs.

As far as drugs are concerned further evidence as to the usefulness of emepronium bromide (Cetiprin) was shown in a recent paper by Brocklehurst et al.[5] Duhar (unpublished) in a double blind trial in normal males given 600 mg. of emepronium bromide showed a delay in onset of desire to void significant of the 5% level, and an increase in bladder volume significant at 1% level. This drug has shown to be similar in its effect to other anticholinergics and no side effects of importance have been reported in elderly people although there have been recent reports of ulceration of the mouth and oesphagus in some younger women taking the drug.[10,11] In using any anticholinergic drug in the treatment of incontinence a precise diagnosis is important to eliminate causes of incontinence other than those which are neurogenic in basis. Once this has been done the drugs must then be given in association with a regime of meticulous nursing in which the patients are taken to the commode or toilet two to four hourly. The drugs probably require to be given for a period of about four weeks in an adequate dosage and of course they must be given at the right time. Incontinence is more often nocturnal than lasting throughout the 24 hours and if this is the case then anticholinergic drugs should be given at 10.00 p.m. and if necessary repeated at 2.00 a.m.

Pads and Appliances

The use of pads and appliances has been the subject of a good deal of study by The Disabled Living Foundation and their publications "Incontinence" and their set of tapes and slides are most useful in the education of nurses and doctors. Perhaps the most interesting development in this field has been the introduction of a gelling pad containing cellulose and colloids which are placed as a powder in a pad similar to an ordinary sanitary pad. When urine is passed into this it forms a jelly which is odourless and which does not wet the skin. This seems a very useful device in the management of occasional wetting. Various workers continue to search for a portable female urinary but so far without success. In the male, Pauls tubing remains as good a standby as any, particularly in males who are paralysed or unconscious.

Three other principles in treatment are now well established but are worth repeating. The first is that any woman reporting incontinence must have an examination of the vulva as well as the rectum. This simplest of procedures is often omitted and, therefore, the cause of the incontinence often misdiagnosed. The second is to emphasise again the importance of an incontinence chart in managing the condition in hospital. The incontinence chart requires adequate nursing with properly trained nurses but this ought to be available in any rehabilitation geriatric ward.

The third is the use of indwelling catheters, which constitute a perfectly rational method of dealing with intractable incontinence in aged women. It must be emphasised that such catheters should be used only on medical advice, that they require proper attention with frequent wash-outs and the use of a proteolytic drug such as Elase and that they should always be used in association with a bag worn on the leg (such as the Bardic Bag) and not one attached to the furniture or lying on the floor.

It is worth noting also that the psychological theory of incontinence in old age propounded by Newman in 1962[18] and based on Sargent's theories in his book "Battle for the Mind" has never been followed up. There is need for some experimental work to substantiate or refute the concept of incontinence in old people have a psychological basis.

Faecal Incontinence

As working classification, that shown in Table 2 is probably the correct one for faecal incontinence. The only part of that classification which might still be regarded as in some doubt is the neurogenic incontinence. Constipation and faecal impaction

Table 2

Causes of faecal incontinence

1.	Symptomatic	– Carcinoma of colon and rectum
		Proctitis
		Diverticular disease
		Ischaemic colitis
		Diabetes
		Purgative administration
		Rectal prolapse
		Destruction of anal sphincter
2.	Constipation	– Faecal impaction
3.	Neurogenic	

are well known as causes of faecal incontinence and the relationship between faecal impaction and immobility has been well shown by Brocklehurst and Khan.[9] Incontinence due to impaction is thus a particular scourge of long-stay wards. The treatment of this condition is by frequent and mechanical emptying of the lower bowel by the use of enemas. The sodium phosphate disposable enema is acceptable and effective in elderly people. In dealing with constipation or faecal impaction causing incontinence, it is necessary to give these enemas daily to a total of seven to ten days or until there is no faecal return.

The question of the neurogenic cause of faecal incontinence was investigated by Freeman and Brocklehurst[3] who compared rectograms and cystometrograms in a group of elderly patients. The findings in both cases were similar in eight out of ten patients, and these findings also confirm those of Brocklehurst[1] that distension of the rectum in incontinent patients leads to intrinsic contractions of the rectum and in many cases this is followed by extrusion of the distending mass. The neurogenic theory of faecal incontinence therefore is as follows. Following the gastrocolic reflex and the movement of faeces into the rectum there is produced a series of uninhibited intrinsic contractions of the rectum itself and this is associated also with a reflex inhibition of tone in the external anal spincter. A formed stool is passed and the patient is unable to prevent this from happening. This is the type of incontinence that requires treatment with chalk and opium described initially by Jarrett and Exton-Smith.[14]

There is still need for further elucidation of motility patterns in the lower bowel among elderly people particularly those with faecal incontinence. The state of the autonomic nervous plexuses also require investigation particularly in view of Smith's work[21] on the effect of anthracine purgatives in producing destruction of the myoneural plexses.

Conclusion

The most important conclusion to be drawn about the management of either faecal or urinary incontinence is the need for a precise diagnosis. It would be helpful to know whether the use of ancillary investigations such as cystometrograms, micturating cystograms and cystoscopy is likely to have more beneficial effects in the long-term treatment of incontinence. This is only one of the problems to which an answer is still required.

References

1. Brocklehurst, J.C. (1951). Incontinence in old people. Edinburgh, Livingstone.

2. Brocklehurst, J.C. (1971). Dysuria in old age. J. Amer. Ger. Soc., 197, 582.

3. Brocklehurst, J.C. (1972). Faecal incontinence : the problems in old age. Proc. Roy. Soc. Med., 65, 66.

4. Brocklehurst, J.C. (1972). Bladder outlet obstruction in elderly women. Modern Geriatrics, 2, 108.

5. Brocklehurst, J.C. (1973). Textbook of Geriatric Medicine and Gerontology. Livingstone, Edinburgh.

6. Brocklehurst, J.C., Armitage, P. and Jouhar, A.J. (1972). Emepronium bromide in urinary incontinence. Age and Ageing, 1, 152.

7. Brocklehurst, J.C., Dillane, J.B., Griffiths, L.L. and Fry, J. (1968). The prevalence and symptomatology of urinary infection in an aged population. Geront. Clin., 10, 242.

8. Brocklehurst, J.C., Fry, J., Griffiths, L.L. and Kalton, C. (1972). Urinary infection and symptoms of dysuria in women aged 45-64 years : their relevance to similar findings in the elderly. Age and Ageing, 1, 41.

9. Brocklehurst, J.C. and Khan, M. Yunis (1969). A study of faecal stasis in old age and the use of 'Dorbanex' in its prevention. Geront. Clin., II, 293.

10. Habeshaw, T. and Bennett, John R. (1972). Ulceration of mouth due to emepronium bromide. Lancet II, 1422.

11. Hale, J.E. and Barnardo, D.E. (1973). Ulceration of mouth due to emepronium bromide. Lancet, I, 493.

12. Isaacs, B. and Walkey, F.A. (1964). A survey of incontinence in the elderly. Geront. Clin., 6, 367.

13. Isaacs, B., Livingstone, M. and Neville, Y. (1972). Survival of the unfittest. Routledge and Kegan Paul, London and Boston.

14. Jarrett, A.S. and Exton-Smith, A.N. (1960). Treatment of faecal incontinence. Lancet, I, 925.

15 Judge, T.G. (1969). The use of quinoestradol in elderly incontinent women - a preliminary report. Geront. Clin., 11, 159.

16 Milne, J.S., Williamson, J., Maule, M.M. and Wallace, E.T. (1972). Urinary symptoms in older people. Modern Geriatrics, 2, 198.

17 Namir, A. and Middleton, R.P. (1954). Stress incontinence in young nulliparous women. Am. J. Obst., 68, 116.

18 Newman, J.L. (1962). Old folk in wet beds. Brit. Med. J., 1, 1824.

19 Packham, D.A. (1971). The epithelial lining of the female trigone. Brit. J. Urol., 43, 201.

20 Sourander, L.B. (1966). Urinary tract infection in the aged. Epidem. Study Supp. 45 Ann. Med. Int. Fenniae, 55.

21 Smith, B. (1970). Disorders of the myenteric plexus. GUT, 11, 271.

22 Tanner, F.R. (1969). Pelvic muscle dysfunction in urinary incontinence. Physiotherapy, 55, 372.

23 Wollin, L.H. (1969). Stress incontinence in young healthy nulliparous female subjects. J. Urol., 101, 545.

24 Woodburne, R.T. (1961). The sphincter mechanism of the urinary bladder and urethra. Anat. Med., 141, 11.

NEW VIEWS ON STROKE

GEORGE F. ADAMS

Professor
Wakehurst House and Queen's
University, Belfast

A misleading title: like much else in medicine what seems new in relation to strokes may often be ancient. For example the syndrome of transient cerebral ischaemia is thought by many people to be a comparatively recent discovery, but 2,000 years ago Soranus of Ephesus[11] observed the episodic and transitory character of this kind of "paralysis"; 300 years ago Willis[21] recognised and described the significance of the collateral circulation we rely on to avoid it; and it is more than 50 years since J. Ramsey Hunt[12] recommended routine examination of the main arteries in the neck in all patients with cerebrovascular disorders drawing attention to their dynamic nature and describing a variety of related transient cerebral symptoms and diminished functional activity which he called the characteristic picture of cerebral intermittent claudication - analagous to the effects of vascular occlusion in the limbs. "Truth is the daughter of time".

Besides not being entirely new, the views that follow are not entirely about strokes since it seems best to consider these within the total spectrum of cerebrovascular disease in a review such as this.

Origins of Cerebrovascular Disorders

Advances in understanding of pathogenesis of cerebrovascular disease cannot be considered in detail, but some appropriate references are given. There have been five main advances in recent years.

(1) Lesions of the intra-cranial vessels are no longer considered in isolation but always in relation to the cerebral circulation as a whole, taking proper account of the large vessels in the neck - the extra-cranial component, including cardiac efficiency in maintaining an adequate head of blood pressure.

(2) Collateral safeguards of the cerebral circulation are recognised to be much more extensive and even more efficient than were supposed.

(3) It is appreciated that collateral circulation is impaired often by disorders which were extrinsic to the blood vessels such as cervical spondylosis, with disc degeneration and exostoses, cervical glands; or intrinsic such as congenital anomalies and arterial disease; above all by the kinks, the narrowing, and the predisposition to thrombosis and embolism associated with atherosclerosis. When many vessels are abnormal blood flow in the territory of some vessels may be cut down to such precarious levels that even very slight changes in the constancy of the supply, or of its composition, may reduce circulation or oxygenation of the dependent parts of the brain below critical minimal need. This is the state of impending cerebral ischaemia described by Corday, Rothenberg and

Tracy[9] as cerebral vascular insufficiency. "Thus although a man is as old as his arteries, he is as young as his collateral circulation will permit".[6]

(4) Some fall-out of cerebral cortical cells, or thinning of the neuraxis is seen as an inevitable consequence of ageing. It reduces the flexibility or adaptability of the older person. This process may be accelerated in ischaemic areas of brain tissue which then become abnormal in that symptoms and signs of disordered function appear quickly in response to relatively slight degrees of oxygen or other metabolic deprivation.

The important contributory factors in this are that:

(a) Even under normal conditions the brain is less able than other organs in the body to withstand ischaemia.

(b) Brain metabolism is highly dependent on the efficient performance of other systems - respiratory, cardiac, renal, hepatic, endocrine and haemopoietic.

Hence the nervous system is easily the most sensitive indicator of disordered function anywhere in the body.[8] Allison[6] underlines this in his comment that although many old people appear to be in excellent health because they have good hearts and collateral circulations, they are none the less fragile. Preservation of the constancy of their internal environment - the milieu interieur of Claude Bernard, is precarious, and they must be "handled with care".

(5) There are many variables, "ischaemia modifying factors"[4] which may act singly or together to produce such symptoms. They include disorders which cause changes in blood pressure, the oxygen-carrying capacity of the blood, or in its thrombogenic or thrombolytic properties.

Investigation of blood flow has progressed from the early studies of the properties of blood vessels and linear flow in them, to estimates of total blood flow, and later of regional blood flow, until research is now focussed on the physical, biochemical and pharmacological responses of the micro-circulation in life. This involves cerebral angiography, isotope brain scanning and even more sophisticated techniques of investigation.

Atheroma is the main cause of the complex alterations in blood flow brought about by distortion of blood vessels, by intimal damage initiating thrombosis or haemorrhage, or by the release of platelet microemboli.

Finally, disorders of cerebral circulation may arise from changes in the composition and quality of the blood including oxygen, carbon-dioxide and glucose content; blood lipid levels, mechanisms of thrombogenesis and thrombolysis; causes of haemoconcentration; altered viscosity, platelet aggregation and adhesiveness; better knowledge of these will extend the development and possibilities of drugs which may be used to improve blood flow.

From consideration of cerebral function in relation to all these aspects of the physiology and pathology of the cerebral circulation, we arrive at the concept of "poverty of reserve" - the state of reduced collateral supply and eroded fail-safe systems which leave the brain at the mercy of even slight impairment or imbalance of factors only indirectly related to the cerebral blood supply. When these factors act, they elicit signs of disordered cerebral function of a kind which depends on the area of brain subjected to the greatest impact of circulatory insufficiency, although this may be remote from the apparent source of the trouble.

Syndromes of Cerebrovascular Disease

Clinically cerebrovascular disease presents in four ways: dementia; transient ischaemia; stroke; postural imbalance.

Dementia

Belief in senility conditioned by faulty cerebral plumbing dies hard, but there is no pathological or physiological evidence to support the theory that the widespread degeneration of nerve cells and tracts found in dementia in old age results from ischaemia caused by atheromatosis.[7] Indeed it seems more likely that parenchymatous degeneration in the grey matter comes first; reduced O_2 tension and blood flow follow in a diffuse slowly progressive process in which atheroma and anoxia play no part.[16]

Defective plumbing may have little to do with dementia but it has much to do with confusion, which so often accompanies illness in old age. This is because the brain is such a sensitive indicator of oxygen deprivation, a good illustration of "poverty of reserve".

Confusion probably appears in patients whose cerebral ischaemia provokes or accentuates the signs of an incipient or overt dementia attributable to other causes.

In practice the essentials are:

(a) To appreciate that phases of mental clouding or confusion may be the first signs of previously unrecognised organic brain disease in elderly patients.

(b) To recognise that mental deterioration is a common associate of cerebrovascular disease and that it is easy to be misled by it in examination or assessment of old people.[5]

(c) In patients with focal signs and confusion to inquire if the mental change preceded the stroke or accompanied it and what was the former mental state.

(d) To be cautious with prognosis of confusion or depression in old people because initial improvement in response to treatment of either may only reveal an underlying intractable dementia.

Transient Ischaemia

Although the distinctions between carotid and vertebral-basilar insufficiency syndromes are now well-recognised, some points relating to transient cerebral ischaemia are not:

(a) The significance of drop attacks as a cause of geriatric disability is still not always appreciated as it should be.

(b) The overall prognosis of transient ischaemia is poor, and for carotid insufficiency is worse than for vertebral basilar ischaemia.

(c) Vertigo, visual disturbances or drop attacks attributable to vertebral basilar ischaemia will continue for a long time without the appearance of permanent neurological deficit. Transient hemiparesis will soon be followed by a stroke.

(d) Early detection of transient ischaemia is important in prediction of strokes; in five years thereafter one-third will have crippling or lethal strokes, one-third will have continuing attacks with or without improvement; and only one-third show spontaneous remission.[20]

(e) Besides the factors which may provoke ischaemia investigation should include a search for:
- (i) Hypertension: ischaemic heart disease: abnormal cardiac rhythm.
- (ii) Hypotension.
- (iii) Temporary shunts - pulses and B.P. in <u>both</u> arms.
- (iv) Sources of thrombosis or embolism.
- (v) Anaemia: polycythaemia.
- (vi) Transient hypoglycaemia.

Strokes

Two groups of patients presenting with strokes have been described:[1,17]

(a) Those where further progress is punctuated by recurrences leading to early death.

(b) Those who survive for many years with few further attacks.

Acheson and Hutchinson[1] believe that multiple strokes are a phenomenon of an "active" form of vascular disease which may be determined by hypertension and our findings[19] may lend support to this view.

Besides the classical arterial syndromes it is possible to recognise:

(a) Non-dominant hemisphere infarction with dense residual hemianopia, hemiplegia or hemianaesthesia accompanied by anosognosia, persistent incontinence and poor prognosis.

(b) Dominant hemisphere transitory ischaemia leading to minimal apraxia (Petren gait)[10]

(c) Anterior cerebral artery infarction resulting in more severe impairment of leg than arm, persistent urinary incontinence (when the non-dominant hemisphere is affected), and personality changes.

(d) Bilateral posterior cerebral artery occlusion[23] causing visual hallucinations, spatial disorientation, occipital blindness and confused behaviour.

Amongst advances relating to established strokes are those which have promoted interest in the treatment of associated intellectual handicaps or mental barriers.[2] They can be classified in four groups:

(i) Impaired learning ability - clouded consciousness; aphasia; memory defects; dementia.

(ii) Disturbed awareness of self or space - with attitudes towards illness disordered by separation from reality (anosognosia; neglect or denial of ownership of hemiplegic limbs; disordered spatial orientation).

(iii) Disordered integrative action (impaired postural function; apraxia; agnosia; perseveration; synkinesia).

(iv) Disturbed emotional behaviour (emotional instability; apathy; loss of confidence; fear; unwillingness to try; catastrophic reactions; depression).

Some of these features are common complications of strokes, but they are not usually mentioned in standard descriptions of management. Patients seldom complain of them being unaware of their difficulties, unable to analyse them, or unable to communicate them, and it is usually an observant attendant who draws attention to the handicap, or it is discovered by a doctor searching for a cause of failure to progress. Identification of these barriers is of practical rather than academic importance because early recognition is necessary if patients are to have the sympathetic understanding and help necessary to find their way round such barriers.

Investigation of mental capacity is only one of the factors applied to the assessment of the prospects of hemiplegic patients. Details of this estimate of "rehabilitation potential" are given elsewhere.[13,14] The essentials[3] are:

Exercise tolerance: making allowance for weakness, stiffness, cardiac or respiratory insufficiency, reaction to drugs.

Motivation: taking account of level of consciousness, ability to communicate, memory, behaviour and performance.

Motor deficit: weakness, spasticity, contracture. Emphasis on restoring mobility of proximal muscle groups, mechanisms of postural control, and a polished walking rhythm; avoiding overuse of the "good" side at the expense of the hemiplegic limbs.

Sensory deficit: including vision, hearing, proprioception, discrimination, cortical integration.

Postural control: the patient who cannot sit with confidence cannot stand, and if he cannot stand reliably he cannot walk. The ability to stand and to walk is conferred by subconscious postural adjustments equivalent to reflex activity including:[18]

(a) mechanisms of postural fixation;
(b) positive supporting reactions and stretch responses of anti-gravity muscles;
(c) righting reactions to counteract gravity or loss of balance;
(d) rhythmical alternating lateral and forward shifts of the centre of gravity involved in body sway to counterpoise the swinging leg.

Inclusion of these in rhythmical movement is a skilled, learned art, not a natural endowment at birth. Proficiency in control of posture, like other achievements of the nervous system, deteriorates with age. Those who were always rather ungainly become more so; even the most polished performers find their skills impaired as they grow older. For a time some make good deficiencies by compensatory tricks devised by conscious or unconscious processes at cortical level, where final integration of movement and associated intellectual activity occurs. Then, when these fail, so does control of posture and movement. This is probably why such disorders arise so readily in old people who have cerebrovascular disease, a condition so commonly related to impaired intellectual function.[15,22].

References

1. Acheson, J. and Hutchinson, E.C. (1971). The natural history of focal cerebral vascular disease. Quart. J. Med., 40, 15.

2. Adams, G.F. and Hurwitz, L.J. (1963). Mental barriers to recovery from strokes. Lancet, 2, 533.

3. Adams, G.F. (1971). Capacity after stroke. Brit. Med. J., 1, 91.

4. Adams, R.D. (1958). Recent developments in cerebrovascular disease. Brit. Med. J., 1, 785.

5. Allison, R.S. (1962). The senile brain. London, E. Arnold Ltd.

6. Allison, R.S. (1964). Mental impairment in the aged. Philadelphia, M. Jacobs Ltd.

7. Barr, D.P. (1955). Atherosclerosis and its effects on the cerebral circulation: In: Cerebral Vascular Diseases. Ed. Wright, I.S. and Luckey, E.H., p. 71. New York. Grune and Stratton Inc.

8. Bedford, P.D. (1959). General medical aspects of confusional states in elderly people. Brit. Med. J., 2, 185.

9. Corday, E., Rotherberg, S.F. and Tracey, J.P. (1953). Cerebral vascular insufficiency. A.M.A. Arch. Neurol. Psychiat., 69, 551.

10. Critchley, M. (1931). The neurology of old age. Lancet, 1, 1121.

11. Drabkin, I.E. (1950). Caelius Aurelianus on acute diseases and on chronic diseases. Chicago, University Press.

12. Hunt, J.R. (1914). The role of the carotid arteries in the causation of vascular lesions of the brain. Amer. J. Med. Sci., 147, 704.

13. Hurwitz, L.J. (1966). Physiotherapy, 338.

14. Hurwitz, L.J. and Adams, G.F. (1972). Rehabilitation of hemiplegia; Indices of assessment and prognosis. Brit. Med. J., 1, 94.

15. Kramer, M. (1958). Sitting, standing and walking. B.M.J., 2, 63.

16 Lassen, N.A. (1961). Studies of internal jugular blood in cerebrovascular disease. Neurology, 11, 41.

17 Marshall, J. and Shaw, D.A. (1959). The natural history of cerebrovascular disease. Brit. Med. J., 1, 1614.

18 Martin, J.P. (1967). The basal ganglia and posture. London, Pitman.

19 Merrett, J.D. and Adams, G.F. (1966). Comparison of mortality rates in elderly hypertensive and normotensive hemiplegic patients. Brit. Med. J., 2, 802.

20 Millikan, C.H. (1966). Diagnosis of the stroke-prone patient.

21 McHenry, L.C. (1969). Garrison's history of neurology. Springfield, Illinois. Thomas.

22 Sheldon, J.H. (1965). Falls in old age. Medicine in Old Age, 199. Pitman, London.

23 Symonds, C. and Mackenzie, I. (1957). Bilateral loss of vision from cerebral infarction. Brain, 80, 415.

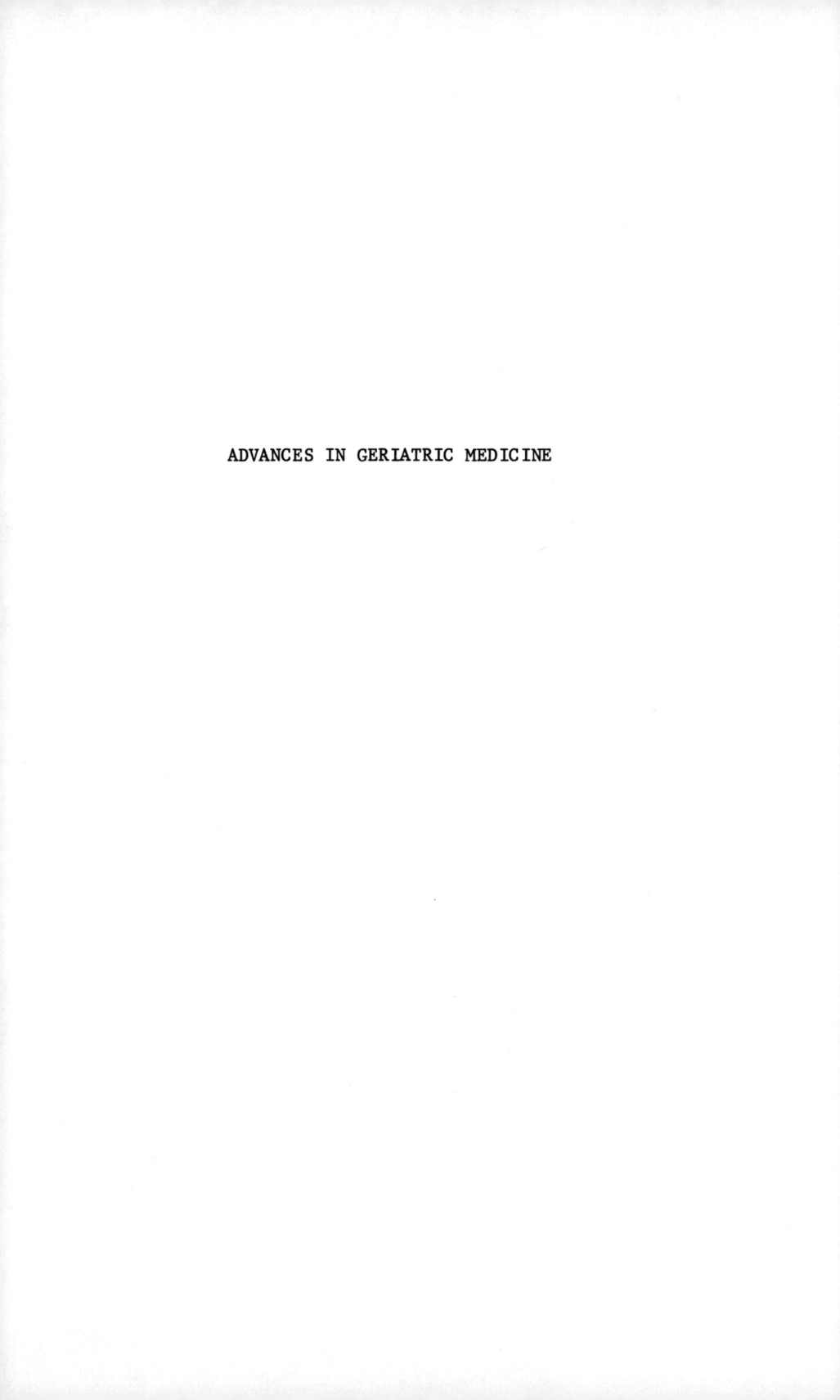

ns IN GERIATRIC MEDICINE

ADVANCES IN GERIATRIC MEDICINE

Chairman's Remarks

JOHN DALL

Consultant Physician
Victoria Geriatric Unit, Glasgow

Ladies and Gentlemen, this afternoon session is devoted to advances in therapeutics, and the speakers will deal with particular systems. I propose in these opening remarks to discuss the wider aspects of drug therapy in the elderly. The physician in geriatric medicine and the general practitioners are well aware that the 'elderly' as a group are, more than any other, likely to present multiple pathologies, and for this reason polypharmacy is common. It is for this very reason that we must be aware of the dangers inherent in prescribing combinations of drugs for outpatients. There are several rules to be borne in mind.

1. Administration

Complex regimes requiring 6 or 7 drugs taken in a variety of schedules from 3 times per week to 4 times daily are unlikely to be successfully achieved outside hospital, and any therapeutic regime must be as simple as treatment will allow.

2. **Absorption**

Many sophisticated, encapsulated preparations are unsuited to elderly who have low gastric acid secretion and may be unable to break down the capsule. Syrup and suspension formulations are easier to take and more likely to be absorbed. Drugs which interfere with Gut motility, e.g., the anticholinergic drugs - widely used in the elderly for Parkinsonism, for bowel and bladder upset, will vary the rate of passage of other preparations through the absorptive area of the bowel and accordingly may enhance the completeness of absorption when prescribed concurrently with other drugs, or may reduce the effective absorption if the anticholinergic drug is then stopped, thus causing the therapeutic effect of the other drug to vary and be suboptimal.

3. **Activity**

The activity of many drugs in common use depends on the amount of 'free' drug in the serum, rather than the total dose, much of which is either protein-bound or tissue-bound, e.g., warfarin is 98% protein-bound and the therapeutic effect is achieved by 2% of the dose. Any alteration in protein-binding will have a considerable effect on the available 'free' warfarin. It is convenient to use warfarin as a research tool in this respect, but we must assume that other drugs which are largely protein-bound behave in the same manner.

(a) Experimental work with plasma dilutions has shown that by the time a dilution of $\frac{1}{2}$ is reached, protein-binding is severely affected and the amount of 'free' drug greatly increased. In a therapeutic situation this would mean side-effects and toxic symptoms from 'normal' drug dosages. Patients with malnutrition, chronic liver disease and chronic renal disease may not show plasma dilutions of $\frac{1}{2}$ as in experiments, but nevertheless, the serum albumin is low and protein-binding impaired.

(b) Competition between drugs for binding sites on protein occurs and many drugs in common use are implicated. With this situation, binding is less efficient and more 'free' drug is available. In practice where exact dosage is necessary and treatment is on a long-term or maintenance basis, e.g., anticoagulant therapy or oral hypoglycaemic agents, the addition of a competing drug to the therapeutic regime is an indication for reduction in maintenance dosage. Sulphonamides and antirheumatic preparations, especially Phenylbutazone, are the principle sources of trouble.

4. Alterations in the 'Milieu Interieur'
(a) Even if the protein-binding of warfarin is not upset, addition of a broad spectrum antibiotic, which sterilizes the gut, reduces symthesis of Vitamin K by flora, destroys the therapeutic balance. Similarly a maintenance dose of digoxin may become a toxic dose if depletion of potassium results from diuretic therapy.

(b) Changes in the rate of metabolic handling of drugs may occur as a result of enzyme induction - but since phenobarbitone is the main enzyme inducer, and this is not in common use in the elderly, enzyme induction is less important than enzyme inhibition. In this context the danger of monoamine oxidase inhibition has been well documented, and since alternatives exist these drugs are better avoided.

5. Excretion
Excretion of drugs via the kidney is affected in two ways:
(a) An overall fall in renal function will delay clearance of the drug and cause serum levels to rise.
(b) Variation in the pH of the urine, a fact well appreciated in the early days of Sulphonamides, may expedite clearance (with loss of therapeutic control) or impair it, resulting in side effects.

In summary, it is this elderly group of patients with diabetes, urinary infections, hypertension and cardiac failure, or chronic bronchitis, osteoarthritis and Parkinsonism and similar combinations of pathology that the demand for polypharmacy arises. If we are to treat adequately the multitude of symptoms, we must be aware of the interactions of the many groups of drugs in common use, if we do not wish to do as much harm as good. To make therapy safer for the patient, we must have a better understanding of the drugs we are prescribing.

ENDOCRINOLOGY IN THE ELDERLY

MICHAEL F. GREEN

Consultant Physician in Geriatric Medicine
The Royal Free Hospital, London

Some of the advances in endocrinology generally, and particularly the introduction of newer methods of investigation, are important in reviewing hormonal function in old age.

Radio-immuno assays have revolutionised the identification and measurement of known hormones, and helped discover new ones, even when plasma concentrations are as low as 3 ng/100 mls. (e.g. free thyroxine). Urinary hormone assays can be helpful, especially in assessing glandular function over a period of time, but diagnosis in the elderly should usually be based on blood samples, because of possible renal impairment and difficulty in obtaining suitable and comprehensive specimens.

Blood stream transport from production to effector site is still the usual, but not absolute, requisite for acceptance as a hormone. Hormones can be produced in the blood (e.g. the renin-angiotensin system), and in the cells (e.g. dihydrotestosterone production from precursors in androgen responsive cells), as well as by endocrine glands. It has been suggested[66] that classical hormones are "first messengers", which activate the adenyl cyclase system located on the inner surface of target cell membranes, catalysing the conversion of A.T.P. to the "second messenger", cyclic AMP. This ubiquitous chemical carries the hormonal message to that cell's messenger R.N.A., and genetic transcription and translation produce a specific metabolic response. This may include the production of another hormone, the "third messenger", such as the steroid hormones of the gonads produced in response to pituitary gonadotrophins.

Prostaglandins may also be "second messengers"[13] particularly involved in defensive reactions in cells. The discovery that prostaglandin synthesis is blocked by aspirin and other non-steroidal anti-inflammatory agents, suggest an exciting field for collaborative research between endocrinologists and geriatric physicians, not only into arthritis but into all "excessive" inflammatory reactions. Horton[35] has reviewed the background physiology.

The hypothalamic-pituitary area is very vascular but it is surprising how few endocrine abnormalities of the hypothalamus and pituitary have been described in the elderly, because as McKeown[50] points out, vascular and degenerative disease of the C.N.S. is very common in old people. Assay of releasing hormones will be a powerful tool in the diagnosis of diseases of hypothalamus, pituitary, and its target organs.[46] It is also surprising that the well maintained production of gonadotrophins into extreme old age (personal observations), in response to gonadal target organ failure, has not been found to produce reactive pituitary changes - the equivalent of secondary and tertiary hyperparathyroidism. One interesting anecdote concerns gonadotrophins: Burckhardt et al.[11] described a highly significant reduction of urinary FSH in elderly women treated with digitalis, compared with untreated controls, giving a possible explanation of the occasional oestrogen-like effect of digoxin in causing gynaecomastia in elderly men.

Dynamic function tests in fit elderly people have not shown any evidence of deteriorating hypothalamic pituitary function[12,30] although there are some conflicting results concerning the maintenance of the normal nyctohemeral (circadian) pituitary-adrenal rhythm in the elderly, possibly caused by sleep disturbances.[57,7,24,56] Personal observation has confirmed that some elderly people in-patients, whose pituitary adrenal axis was being studied during a 24-hour period, did show disturbed sleep patterns. Depression is also associated with abnormalities of sleep and with abnormal pituitary-adrenal rhythms,[16] which can also be disturbed in heart failure.[15]

It is becoming increasingly difficult for laboratories to provide a comprehensive endocrine service,[1] and it may be difficult to justify investigations in elderly people, but endocrine abnormalities are certainly being missed, when traditional and newer diagnostic methods might reveal unsuspected diagnoses, and indicate alternative methods of management. TSH assay might be particularly valuable in sorting out hypothyroidism in the elderly.

It is important to emphasise:

1. The majority of significant endocrine pathology in old people is the result of pre-existing conditions, or arises as an inevitable part of the accumulating pathology of a long life.

2. There is a scanty literature concerning endocrine function tests and classical syndromes in the elderly, with the exception of diabetes mellitus (which is reviewed separately in the symposium), the thyroid gland, and the confusing field of bone metabolism.

3. The highest clinical acumen is often necessary in assessing the endocrine status of old people, because of problems of accumulated pathology, the effects of multiple prescribing

on investigations, and because laboratory results are often conflicting.

4. Identification of endocrine disorders in the elderly often justifies energetic management.

THYROID

L thyroxine (T4) is often regarded as the main effective circulating hormone but L-tri-iodothyronine (T3) is probably metabolically even more important than T4[64], and T4 acts partially as a prehormone, being converted to T3 before acting on its target cells.[65] T3 thyrotoxicosis has been described by Wahner[71], usually with toxic nodular goitres, and patients with low PBI's after thyroidectomy can have euthyroidism maintained almost completely by T3 (personal observation).

Tests

1. <u>Thyroxine index and ratio.</u> Serum protein bound iodine (PBI), and T4 measurements estimate thyroid hormone bound to proteins (TBP), particularly thyroxine-binding-globulin (TBG), and are falsely raised by many drugs which affect protein binding, including iodides (X-ray media and clioquinol - "Enterovioform", CIBA), phenytoin and oestrogens, and decreased by salicylates and in association with severe stresses, including hypothermia. The T3 uptake measures unoccupied TBP sites and falsely hypothyroid results are produced by oestrogens (stibboestrol) and a rise in TBG, hyperthyroid ones by anabolic steroids and a fall in TBG. Since thyroidal status is related to the free thyroxine level, which is usually proportional to the product of PBI (or serum T4) and T3 uptake, abnormalities which confuse thyroid function tests can often be minimised by measuring a PBI/T3 uptake ratio, such as the Free Thyroxine Index (FTI)[36], or the Effective Thyroxine Ratio (ETR).[70]

2. <u>Radio immuno assay.</u> Hypothalamic thyroid-releasing-hormone (TRH), and thyroid stimulating hormone (TSH) assays may

be useful in distinguishing primary and secondary hypothyroidism, and it is interesting how rarely we tend to diagnose hypothyroidism due to pituitary disease in the elderly. In a recent review Evered and Hall[19], divide hypothyroidism into overt (when clinical assessment and investigations are clearly diagnostic, and a hazard such as myxoedema coma could occur), mild (when more insidious symptoms and equivocal test results may give conflicting conclusions) and preclinical (asymptomatic, when reduced thyroidal activity is compensated for by a raised output of TSH). The preclinical group are likely to have circulating thyroid antibodies or hypercholesterolaemia, and may be more susceptible to lipid disorders and ischaemic heart disease than the population generally[22] and can only be identified conclusively by finding an elevated basal TSH level. Serum TSH will always be raised in primary hypothyroidism, and if still raised in treated patients would suggest inadequate therapy.

Hypothyroidism

Incidence. Computerised collation of clinical and biochemical data is now being used for follow-up of treated thyrotoxics and for population surveys[47], and a diagnostic index for hypothyroidism has been developed by Billewicz.[5] Sensitive measurements of target organ function such as the ankle reflex time are not very helpful, as many elderly people have absent ankle jerks, and there is considerable overlap between hypo-, eu-, and hyper-thyroid subjects.

The problem of iatrogenic hypothyroidism following treatment of thyrotoxicosis is very serious; Green and Wilson[31] suggest that radio-iodine therapy is followed at ten years by incidence of hypothyroidism of 35% or more, with an additional annual accruement subsequently; the technique and dosage of radio-iodine administration may reduce the risk, and the risk of surgical treatment may also be less, or thyrotoxicosis recurs. The follow-up of treated thyrotoxic patients should therefore be lifelong, and may become a major cumulative problem in the elderly.

Surveys in the elderly give conflicting results - Lloyd and Goldberg[49] had to rely heavily on clinical judgment; Thomson et al.[69] in a survey of elderly people at home did not find convincing evidence of undiagnosed hypo- or hyper-thyroidism very common, based mainly on PBI measurements. However, Jefferys[38] described an overall incidence of thyroid disease of 5.7% in 317 consecutive patients admitted to a geriatric unit, with PBI and T3 uptakes as initial tests. Additional measurements[39] on a similar group showed that up to 20% of the euthyroid patients had reduced TBG levels; many had reduced serum albumin, and the severity of illness was thought to be the major factor in the reduction of these proteins. The results justify measuring both PBI and T3 uptake (or equivalent) in the elderly suspected of having thyroid abnormalities, with the calculation of an FTI or ETR when indicated, and even of carrying out routine thyroid function tests on every new admission to a geriatric department.

Non-specific observations such as pulse rate, weight, mental test score, ECG, facial photography and voice recordings may be useful before and during a trial of treatment of hypothyroidism, when laboratory results are conflicting.

<u>Clinically</u>. The manifestations of hypothyroidism are protean[45], but it is important to remember that there are few causes of a slow pulse in old age, that perceptive deafness is common in hypothyroidism and improves on treatment, that vitiligo may be a clue to autoimmune disease, and that unexplained croakiness, or cerebellar ataxia[40], may be caused by hypothyroidism. Remediable confusion can easily be ignored, and vague musculoskeletal symptoms such as aching and stiffness, often with paraesthesiae, may dominate the clinical picture.[29]

Only a few cases of "spontaneous" hypothermia are due to hypothyroidism. A low PBI in hypothermic patients may be caused by abnormal proteins[53], and the significance is often counteracted by a proportionately high or high normal T3 uptake. Chlorpromazine is known to contribute to hypothermia, and may partially act by a central effect on TRF release. I have found no evidence of adrenal insufficiency in hypothermic (or other ill elderly) patients, although large doses of hydrocortisone may be justified in treating any severely shocked patient.

Treatment

L-thyroxine is a simple and effective replacement therapy, as long as patients continue to take it, and it is given in appropriate dosage. Most elderly people seem to be restored to euthyroidism by doses not exceeding 0.2 mg a day, starting with 0.025 or 0.05 mg per day and increasing in steps of 0.025 or 0.05 mg every two to three weeks; caution is particularly necessary in those with underlying ischaemic heart disease. Cardiac and respiratory function in response to exercise, of hypothyroid patients of all ages, has been shown to improve after treatment.[10] Individual requirements vary, and two elderly patients have recently been treated with 0.4 and 0.6 mg a day respectively; these dosages were only achieved over many months, but were necessary to restore euthyroidism, and were without side effects. L-tri-iodo-thyroxine is indicated in hypothermic victims judged to be truly hypothyroid, because of its rapidity of action (half-life 1 day; half-life of T4 almost a week). It has no other place in the management of hypothyroidism; there is no advantage in using a combined T3/T4 preparation[59] which can give unpleasant side effects.

THYROTOXICOSIS

The usual clinical features of hyperthyroidism are often modified, or absent, in old people[44], although the classical exophthalmic goitous syndrome does occur. Cardiac symptomatology - atrial fibrillation and congestive cardiac failure and apathy[68,42] with weight loss, depression and confusion may dominate the picture. The success rate of a clinical scoring index[32] is reduced by a tendency to atypicality, and the frequency of mental effects and concurrent dementia. All the cases of thyrotoxicosis discovered in a London geriatric department[42], were atypical and previously undiagnosed, and represented more than 2% of all admissions. Thyrotoxic patients over 60 were half as numerous as those between 45 and 60, attending a Glasgow thyroid clinic.[44]

Although thyroid function tests may be falsely raised by drugs and X-ray media, several of our patients have had raised tests without clinical evidence of hyperthyroidism or discovered the reasons for the laboratory abnormalities. A lengthy follow-up has seen persistence of the slight laboratory abnormalities or a return to normal. Certainly, atypical thyrotoxicosis may only be discovered by routine testing of all patients, or of selected groups, e.g., those with heart failure, AF, and mental symptoms.

The recently described syndrome of T3 thyrotoxicosis[34] can occur in the elderly[38], and raised levels of T3 may herald the onset of conventional hyperthyroidism[4] - it is not yet known how common T3 thyrotoxicosis is at any age. In suspected cases of hyperthyroidism with normal PBI, T3 resin uptake, and radio iodine uptake, non-suppressibility of the gland uptake would suggest T3 toxicosis, if serum T3 levels are unobtainable.

Treatment of Thyrotoxicosis

Anti-thyroid drug treatment with carbimazole is the first choice, as surgery and radio-iodine have such serious complications, particularly subsequent hypothyroidism. It can be supplemented by beta adrenergic blockage in patients with disturbing sympathetic-mediated symptoms including tachycardia;

practolol has proved its worth in treating elderly subjects with supraventricular arrhythmias.[2] Carbimazole treatment can be continued for one to two years and may be followed by cure in up to half the patients[74] or can be continued indefinitely if necessary.

CALCIUM METABOLISM

The aetiology and management of osteoporosis continue to provoke many studies and hypotheses. There are a variety of radiological indices for measuring bone (e.g., Barnett et al[3], Exton-Smith et al.[20]), but it is difficult to select the best method of assessing the inevitable loss of bone that seems to accompany ageing in both sexes and all races.[27] In reviewing the clinical significance and pathogenesis of osteoporosis Nordin[51] describes the occurrence of fractures at different ages: (1) the lower forearm, particularly in women between 50 and 65; (2) proximal femur, in both sexes particularly over 70; and (3) vertebral crushing which can occur at any age, but is commonest in elderly women. He suggests that a slight hypercalciuria occuring postmenopausally causes a significant calcium loss through nocturnal calciuria which is not replaced by dietary intake, and that the lost calcium is released from bone by the decline in oestrogens allowing a partial release of parathormone (PTH) inhibition of bone resorption. The loss might only represent a net daily debit of 15 mg; loss could continue for years, and might also contribute to osteoporosis in men in whom gonadal decline does occur but is later and slower.

Severe osteoporosis can occur in Turner's Syndrome, which is characterised by bodily abnormalities including ovarian agenesis, when the osteoporosis is really congenital and histology usually reveals gross paucity of all bone elements. The fate of these women is uncertain, as they are usually diagnosed young, and lapse from follow-up. It may be that they die in middle age, from pathology partly ascribable to oestrogen lack, such as bone and cardiovascular disease. Contraceptive hormones, and oestrogens used in the treatment of prostatic carcinoma, have worrying side-effects, although there is evidence that oestrogens can prevent or retard demineralisation of bone[17]; short-term benefit has not been seen in a series of oestrogen-treated Turners.[28] Evidence that lack of oestrogen in castrated women is associated with increased susceptibility to coronary heart disease[52] has not lead to general acceptance of oestrogen replacement in oophorectomised or postmenopausal women. As long ago as 1963 Stamler et al.[60] reduced the frequency of recurrence of heart attacks in men, using long-term oestrogen therapy.

The amount of calcified bone taken up in early life[63] and dietary lack and poor calcium and vitamin D absorption in later life, are probably the most important factors in determining bone mass, although osteoporosis is likely to be multi-factorial. The lack of exposure to sunlight in the housebound elderly, and diminished muscle action on periosteum may be more important than we realise. Deficient body collagen may be a factor in causing osteoporosis, and it has been suggested[6] that androgen therapy may be indicated in the treatment of osteoporosis in women. Although gross malabsorption states may be correctable Nordin[51] suggests that vitamin D supplements should be given to all elderly people, to prevent the pronounced fall in calcium absorption of normal over eighties, noted by Bullamore et al.[9] This calcium malabsorption, when combined with oestrogen-deficient urinary calcium loss, could eventually lead to osteoporosis, as well as osteomalacia, in susceptible individuals; The D.H.S.S. recommendation of 100 IU of supplemental vitamin D a day might be insufficient for this purpose. The place of other supplements in preventing or treating osteoporosis is uncertain but high calcium and protein intakes, fluoride[43], and vitamin C[62], have been advocated singly or in combination with each other and with oestrogens and androgens.

Hypercalcaemia

This is a fairly common finding in the course of multiple biochemical screening, and the causes are virtually the same as those for younger people, including the various forms of true and pseudo-hyperparathyroidism, excessive vitamin D and/or calcium intake (including iatrogenic administration) vitamin D hypersensitivity, bone diseases, and neoplasia. It is commonly associated with immobilisation, and a serum calcium measurement should be considered in every patient with one of these disorders, if not in every old person admitted to hospital. Hypercalcaemia causes vague symptoms of weakness, anorexia, nausea, constipation, nocturia, confusion, major psychoses, and even death. Corneal calcification is a sign which can be confirmed using a hand lens in strong tangential light.[72]

It is sometimes difficult to discover the reason for high (and low) serum calcium values, even after correcting for protein binding abnormalities. Although hypercalcaemia can produce so much morbidity, and some of these cases may have hyperparathyroidism, exploration of the neck is not always justified.

Osteomalacia

Altered calcium metabolism due to anticonvulsants[37] is caused by induction of hepatic microsomal enzymes, resulting in increased vitamin D requirements. This requirement may be higher than the usual intakes, and has been found to cause osteomalacia in younger people.

Renal Disease

The incidence of renal impairment rises with increasing age, and kidney disease is often associated with disturbed calcium metabolism. The kidney secretes the hormonal metabolite of vitamin D1, 25 dihydroxycholicalciferol (1,25-DHCC)[23] which is more important than vitamin D in the control of gut and bone calcium transfer. Parathormone may suppress the hydroxylation of 25 hydroxycholicalciferol (25 HCC) to 1,25-DHCC by direct renal action.[26] This may partly explain the complex calcium chemistry of both renal and parathyroid disease - severe bone disease in chronic renal failure could be due to high levels of circulating PTH interfering with vitamin D metabolism.

Pagets Disease and Calcitonin

Hypercalcaemia is rare in Pagets, and response to therapy is usually judged by relief of bone pain and reduction of serum alkaline phosphatase. Success in the long-term should be visible radiologically. The RNA synthesis-blocker mithramycin has been reported to diminish bone pain[14] as have diphosphonate[58] and calcitonin.[61] Calcitonin is produced by the non-thyroxine producing C cells of the thyroid, and is thought to act mainly by inhibiting bone absorption. Calcitonin also has a possible role in treating hypercalcaemia associated with malignancy[41], and even in treating osteoporosis - experimental evidence supports this view.[25]

NEOPLASTIC DISEASE

Endocrine and metabolic abnormalities should be considered in all elderly people with neoplasia or bizzarre clinical and biochemical presentations; Ross[55] has recently reviewed the subject. "Ectopic" secretion may produce hormones indistinguishable from the naturally-occurring chemical, or biological equivalents. Syndromes include the production of corticotrophin, parathormone, vasopressin, gonadotrophins, melanophore-stimulating hormone, gastrin, and hypoglycaemia. These syndromes have most commonly been described in association with oat cell carcinoma of the bronchus[54], and may be multiple.

Syndrome of Inappropriate Secretion of Anti-diuretic Hormone (SIADH)

This has been described with various diseases, including bronchial carcinoma, tuberculosis, pneumonia, head injuries, cerebral tumours, and myxoedema.[48] There may be tumorous production of ADH, or inappropriate pituitary secretion in response to changes in intravascular fluids and extracellular osmolality. The inappropriate ADH causes water retention, hyponatraemia, natriuresis, and a drop in body fluid osmolality. Suspicion is aroused in the presence of neoplasia and/or hyponatraemia, with symptoms of anorexia, nausea, vomiting, and excitation and/or depression followed by lethargy with convulsions and coma. Fluid sodium may be as low as 100 to 110 mEQ/L with a low urea and osmolality, and with an abnormally increased urinary sodium loss, the urine becomes hypertonic compared to plasma. There may be a renal tubular defect with glycosuria and amino-aciduria. There will usually be raised levels of circulating ADH. The differential diagnosis is from hyponatraemia associated with congestive cardiac failure or hepatic cirrhosis when oedema is usually present, and from adrenal insufficiency. Treatment is by fluid deprivation, treatment of the underlying disease if possible and sometimes fludrocortisone.

Growth Hormone

Although the hypophysectomised adult does not apparently need H.G.H. replacement, polypeptides from the pituitary derived from H.G.H. may contribute to the development of diabetes mellitus by causing both early hypoglycaemia, and late hyperglycaemia.[8] The discovery that the release of a sulphation factor affecting bone, and probably cartilage development, called somatomedin, is stimulated by H.G.H. may lead to the discovery of important effects in geriatric physiology.[67]

Three new cases of active acromegaly have been diagnosed in our routine geriatric practice during the last three years. The diagnosis has been confirmed by raised H.G.H. levels which have not suppressed during an oral glucose tolerance test. None had other conditions which can cause paradoxical elevation of H.G.H., such as cerebral tumour, uraemia and heart failure.[33]

Luckily they did not have evidence of visual defects or hypertension, and although two had diabetic GTT's the only diabetic management necessary was dietary, and none required pituitary ablation.

AGEING

Virtually any glandular abnormality can occur in the over 65's. The carcinoid syndrome has recently been described in an 80-year old[21], and we have recently unsuccessfully treated a woman of 85 who had heart failure and thyrotoxicosis due to a functioning carcinomatous thyroid nodule. Although gonadal function declines with age, and the general social climate is against sexual relationships in old age, there is no reason why happy and satisfactory relationships may not be continued into extreme old age. Gonadal replacement therapy has not been proved to restore youth to those who are aged.

Although it may be possible to modify major causes of morbidity and mortality such as osteoporosis and arteriosclerosis by hormonal treatment, there is no evidence that physiological or pathological ageing are caused by glandular disorders. Endocrine abnormalities do occur in premature ageing syndromes, such as progeria, Werner's syndrome[73], and in mothers of children with Down's syndrome[18], but are not apparently the cause of the abnormal senescence in these patients.

References

1. Anderson, J., Bagshawe, K.D., Black, D.A.J., Granstom, W.I., Fowler, P.B.S., Ledingham, J.M., Lee, J., Morris, N., Milne, M.D., Wardener, H.E. de, Wrong, O.M. and Wyman, A.L. (1972). Lancet, 1, 95.

2. Ashton, F. (1970). Geront. clin., 12, 321.

3. Barnett, E.C., Nordin, B.E.C. (1960). Clin. Radio., 11, 166.

4. Bellabarba, D. (1972). Clin. Res., 20, 421.

5. Billewicz, W.Z., Chapman, R.S., Crooks, J., Day, M.E., Gossage, J., Wayne, E.J. and Young, J.A. (1969). Quart. J. Med., 38, 225.

6. Black, M.M., Shuster, S. and Bottoms, E. (1970). Brit. Med. J., 4, 773.

7. Blichert-Toft, M. (1971). Geront. clin., 13, 215.

8. Bornstein, J., Krahl, M.E., Mashall, L.B., Gould, M.K. and Armstrong, J. McD. (1968). Biochemica et Biophysica Acta, 156, 31.

9. Bullamore, J.R., Gallagher, J.C., Wilkinson, R., Nordin, B.E.C. and Marshall, D.H. (1970). Lancet, 2, 535.

10. Burack, R., Edwards, R.H.T., Green, M.F. and Jones, N.L. (1971). Journ. Pharmacol. and Exp. Therap., 1, 212.

11. Burckhardt, D., Vera, C.A. and LaDue J.S. (1968). Ann. Int. Med., 65, 1069.

12. Cartlidge, N.E.F., Black, M.M., Hall, M.R.P. and Hall, R. (1970). Geront. clin., 12, 65.

13. Collier, H.O.J. (1971). Nature, 232, 17.

14. Condon, J.R., Reith, S.B.M., Nassim, J.R., Millard, F.J.C., Hilb, A. and Stainthorpe, E.M. (1971). Brit. Med. J., 1, 421.

15. Connolly, M. and Wills, M. (1967). Brit. Med. J., 2, 25.

16. Conroy, R.T.W.L., Hughes, B.D. and Mills, J.N. (1968). Brit. Med. J., 3, 405.

17. Davis, M.E., Lanzi, L.H. and Cox, A.B. (1970). Obstet. and Gynec., 36, 187.

18. Emanuel, I., Milham, S. Jr., Sever, L.E. and Thuline H.C. (1972). Lancet, 2, 361.
19. Evered, D. and Hall, R. (1972). Brit. Med. J., 1, 290.
20. Exton-Smith, A.N., Millard, P.H., Payne, P.R. and Wheeler, E.F. (1969). Lancet, 2, 1153.
21. Fisher, R.H. and Hussain, S.M.A. (1971). Geront. clin., 6, 368.
22. Fowler, P.B.S., Swale, J. and Andrews, H. (1970). Lancet, 2, 488.
23. Fraser, D.R. and Kodicek, E. (1970). Nature, 228, 764.
24. Friedman, M., Green, M.F. and Sharland, D.E. (1969). Journ. Geront., 24, 292.
25. Fujita, T., Orimo, H., Ohata, M., Yoskikawa, M., Nakanishi, K. and Misaka, E. (1968). Endocr. Ja., 15, 8.
26. Galante, L., Colston, K., Macauley, S. and Macintyre, I. (1972). Lancet, 1, 985.
27. Garn, S.M. (1970). The Earlier Gain and Later Loss of Cortical Bone. Springfield, Illinois.
28. Ginsberg, J. (1972). Personal communication.
29. Golding, D.N. (1970). Ann. Rheum. Dis., 29, 10.
30. Green, M.F. and Friedman, M. (1968). Geront. clin., 10, 334.
31. Green, M. and Wilson, G.M. (1964). Brit. Med. J., 1, 1005.
32. Hall, R., Amos, J. and Ormston, R.J. (1971). Brit. Med. J. 1, 582.
33. Hartog, M. and Wright, A.D. (1972). Brit. J. Hosp. Med., April, 853.
34. Hollander, C.S., Mitsuma, T., Nihei, N., Skenkman, L., Burday, S.Z. and Blum, M. (1972). Lancet, 1, 609.
35. Horton, E.W. (1969). Physiol. Reviews, 49, 122.
36. Howorth, P.J.N. and Maclagan, N.F. (1969). Lancet, 1, 224.
37. Hunter, J., Maxwell, J.D., Stewart, D.A., Parsons, V. and Williams, R. (1971). Brit. Med. J., 4, 202.
38. Jefferys, P.M. (1972). Age and Ageing, 1, 33.
39. Jefferys, P.M., Farran, H.E.A., Hoffenberg, R., Fraser, P.M. and Hodkinson, H.M. (1972). Lancet, 2, 924.
40. Jellinek, E.H. and Kelly, R.E. (1960). Lancet, 2, 225.

41 Kammerman, S. and Canfield, R.E. (1970). J. Clin. Endocrinol. Metab., **31**, 70.

42 Kendall-Taylor, P. (1972). Brit. Med. J., **2**, 337.

43 Kuhlencordt, F., Kruse, H.P., Lozano-Tinkin, C. and Eckermeier, L. (1970). Fluoride in Medicine, Ed. Thomas L. Vischer.

44 Lazarus, J.H., Harden, R. McG. (1969). Geront. clin., **11**, 371.

45 Leader (1970). Brit. Med. J., **2**, 61.

46 Leader (1972). Brit. Med. J., **1**, 66.

47 Leader (1972). Brit. Med. J., **1**, 457.

48 Leader (1972). Brit. Med. J., **3**, 489.

49 Lloyd, W.H. and Goldberg, I.J.L. (1961). Brit. Med. J., **2**, 1256.

50 McKeown, F. (1965). Pathology of the Aged, p. 308. Butterworths, London.

51 Nordin, B.E.C. (1971). Brit. Med. J., **1**, 571.

52 Robinson, R.W., Higano, N., Cohen, W.D. (1960). New. Engl. J. Med., **263**, 828.

53 Rosin, A.J. and Exton-Smith, A.N. (1964). Brit. Med. J., **1**, 16.

54 Ross, E.J. (1968). Recent Advances in Endocrinology. Ed. James V.H.T., 8th edition, Churchill, London.

55 Ross, E. (1972). Medicine, **2**, 125.

56 Serio, M., Piolanti, P., Roman, S., De Magistris, L. and Guisti, G. (1970). Journ. Geront., **25**, 95.

57 Silverberg, A., Rizzo, F. and Krieger, D.T. (1968). J. Clin. Endocr. and Metab., **28**, 1662.

58 Smith, R., Russell, R.G.G. and Bishop, M. (1971). Lancet, **1**, 945.

59 Smith, R.N., Taylor, S.A. and Massey, J.C. (1970). Brit. Med. J., **4**, 145.

60 Stamler, J. et al. (1963). J. Amer. med. Ass., **183**, 632.

61 Stamler, J., Pick, R., Katz, L.N., Pick, A., Kaplan, B., Berkson, D.M. and Century, D. (1963). J. Amer. med. Ass., **183**, 632.

62 Stein, L. and Beller, M.L. (1970). Geriatrics, **25**, No.3, 159.

63 Sterart R.J.C., Sheppard, H.C., Preece, R.F. and Exton-Smith, A.N. (1972). Age and Ageing, 1, 1.

64 Sterling, K. (1970). Rec. Prog. Horm. Res., 26, 249.

65 Sterling, K., Bellabarba, D., Newman, E.S., Bremmer, M.A.J. (1969). J. Clin. Invest., 48, 1150.

66 Sutherland, E.W., Oye, I. and Butcher, R.W. (1965). Prog. Rec. Horm. Res., 21, 623.

67 Tanner, J.M. (1972). Nature, 237, 433.

68 Thomas, F.B., Mazzaferri, E.L. and Skillman, T.F. (1970). Ann. Inter. Med., 72, 679.

69 Thomson, J.A., Andrews, G.R., Caird, F.I. and Wilson, R. (1972). Age and Ageing, 1, 158.

70 Thorson, S.C., Mincey, E.K., McIntosh, H.W. and Morrison, R.T. (1972). Brit. Med. J., 2, 67.

71 Wahner, H.W. and Gorman, C.A. (1971). New Engl. J. Med., 284, 225.

72 Watson, L. (1972). Medicine, 2, 148.

73 Wells, R.S. (1972). Proc. Roy. Soc. Med., 65, 525.

74 Wilson, G.M. (1967). Symposium Thyroid Disease and Calcium Metabolism, p. 51-76. Royal College of Physicians, Edinburgh.

PARKINSONISM

FRANCIS I. CAIRD

Senior Lecturer in Geriatric Medicine
University of Glasgow

Parkinsonism is an important condition in its own right in geriatric medicine, because it is a not infrequent cause of severe disability. It is also an area of geriatric neurology in which there have been major advances in recent. years. These advances consist of an important change in thought about aetiology, a clearer idea of prevalence, and a revolution in therapy.

In the past, Parkinsonism in the elderly has often been thought to be of vascular or arteriosclerotic aetiology, but in recent years there has been increasing agreement among neurologists that 'arteriosclerotic Parkinsonism' is very rare, or even non-existent.[13] Indeed if one looks at elderly patients with Parkinsonism with an unbiased eye, and does not assume that evidence of arteriosclerosis elsewhere automatically implies an arteriosclerotic cause of brain disease, it is very difficult to see any great neurological difference from middle-aged patients with the same condition. The same three cardinal features, tremor, rigidity, and bradykinesia, are all present, though tremor tends to be less marked, and rigidity and bradykinesia to predominate. To the extent that arteriosclerotic Parkinsonism is thought to differ from the idiopathic type, and to have different prognostic and therapeutic implications, then the realisation that it is very rare may well remove an obstacle to thought and to correct treatment. This is an advance.

The prevalence of Parkinsonism has been reported as 6 per 1000 people aged 65 or more,[5] and as 15 per 1000.[11] Our own observations in Glasgow, based on the examination of over 800 people aged 65 or more living at home,[3] show that the latter figure is more nearly correct. The prevalence of 16 per 1000 for Parkinsonism compares with a figure of 166 per 1000 for cerebrovascular disease (cerebral infarction 73 per 1000, transient ischaemic attacks 93 per 1000). One point of substantial interest and no little importance revealed in our study is that the prevalence of essential or 'senile' tremor (often with a striking family history) is virtually identical to that of Parkinsonism in the elderly. The importance of this differential diagnosis is not sufficiently stressed in current teaching. The therapeutic implications require emphasis : essential tremor should not be treated with levodopa.

The revolution in treatment of Parkinsonism which has resulted from the introduction of levodopa and amantadine has been slow to affect the elderly. There is in the literature[2,10,16] the strong impression that elderly patients are unable to tolerate adequate doses of levodopa without a high frequency of side effects, especially neuropsychiatric, necessitating discontinuance of treatment. It is implied that there is doubt whether elderly patients should be treated at all.

In Glasgow, some two years ago, a trial was set up to investigate whether the use of small initial doses of levodopa, with small increments and a low final dose, could give elderly patients with Parkinsonism the benefits of levodopa without an undue risk of side effects.[4] 68 patients from continuing-care wards in 10 hospitals were screened for possible inclusion in the trial, and 21 accepted. There were 17 women and 4 men, aged 68 years or more, in whom Parkinsonism was the principal cause of disability, and none of whom had received phenothiazines. None had a history of an encephalitic illness, and arteriosclerotic Parkinsonism was not diagnosed. Their functional state, their physical signs, and their mental function were assessed before levodopa was begun, and at regular intervals thereafter. Most had gross disability, and initial intellectual impairment was rated as severe in 8, moderate in 7, and mild in 6. Levodopa was begun in a dose of 125 mg. three times a day, and this was increased by 125 mg. every 3-4 days, until a final dose of 1.5-2G was reached. At the same time anticholinergic drugs were gradually withdrawn, over a period of 4-6 weeks.

16 of the 21 patients completed 6 months on levodopa. 3 of the remainder died within the first 9 weeks, none from conditions attributable to treatment. 2 were withdrawn from the trial because of side effects. Of the 16 who completed the trial, 9 showed considerable improvement. 5 were discharged home, an outcome not previously considered possible in 4; 3 of these 5 were initially dependent on help for dressing and walking. In 3 others there was improvement in physical and mental function, with increased independence, decreased disorientation and nocturnal restlessness, and variable improvement in physical signs. In 4 there was no improvement; 3 of these were initially chairfast, and 3 showed severe intellectual impairment.

Semiquantitative measures of physical signs confirmed this general pattern of improvement (Table 1). Tremor, rigidity, and bradykinesia all showed statistically significant change, but speech did not, though increased strength of voice is very often the first clinically detectable evidence of benefit from levodopa. An assessment scale for activities of daily living, based on scores for walking, dressing, feeding and toileting, also showed statistically significant change in the group as a whole (Table 1). There was an improvement in average performance in each of six timed performance tests (rising from a chair, walking 10 yards with one turn, putting on a sock, doing up 3 buttons, writing a sentence of 5 monosyllabic words, and drawing a circle), and several patients unable to carry out the test before therapy became able to do so (Table 2).

The changes in mental function are of great interest. Three tests were used, a modification of the Crichton Geriatric Behavioural Rating Scale,[15] a memory and information test involving orientation, calculation, memory for remote and recent personal events, and a test of recall, and the set test of open-ended questions devised by Akhtar and Isaacs.[1] No demonstrable learning or placebo effects have been found when these tests have been used in other situations. There was a statistically significant improvement in all three tests in the group as a whole (Table 3). No patient showed significant deterioration, either clinically or on testing. There are many possible factors to be taken into account in assessing the meaning of this improvement: mental stimulation due to inclusion in the trial itself, an 'arousal effect' of the drug,[12] improved motor performance, relief of apathy, or change of mood. What is important is that a measurable change in mental function occurred, and that in no case was there demonstrable deterioration.

The side effects encountered were in general relatively slight. Though 13 patients had nausea, with vomiting in 8, in only 2 was this severe enough to cause withdrawal from the trial. 7 patients developed symptomatic orthostatic hypotension while on levodopa; 3 of these had had a significant postural drop of blood pressure (20 mm Hg or more) before therapy. Symptoms were controlled by a small dose reduction or a temporary cessation of dose increments. Overall, the standing systolic blood pressure tended to fall for the first 8-12 weeks, and then to rise almost

Table 1

Changes in physical signs and activities of daily living (A.D.L.). Scores in 16 patients completing 6 months on levodopa.

	Mean Score Before / After 6 months on levodopa		Significance of change*
Tremor	3.0	1.9	< 0.02
Rigidity	7.4	5.0	< 0.01
Bradykinesia	19.9	13.9	< 0.001
A.D.L. Score	6.5	4.3	< 0.01

* P value for Student's test for a paired series.

Table 2

Changes in timed performance tests in 16 patients completing 6 months on levodopa

Test	No. Capable Initially	No. Capable Finally	Mean Time (Secs.) Before†	Mean Time (Secs.) After†	Significance of difference*
Rise from chair	5	9	5.6	2.8	N.S.
Walk 10 yards	7	10	43	20	<0.05
Put on sock	6	9	41	18	<0.001
Do up 3 buttons	9	13	49	28	<0.01
Write 5 words	14	14	55	38	N.S.
Draw a circle	15	16	12	8	N.S.

* P value for Student's test for a paired series.

† for those initially capable of the test.

Table 3

Changes in mental function tests in 16 patients completing 6 months on levodopa

Test	Mean Score Before	After	Significance of Difference*
Behavioural Rating Scale	11.4	14.4	<0.01
Questionnaire	17.5	23.0	<0.001
Set Test	23.0	29.5	<0.02

* P value for Student's test for a paired series.

to pre-treatment levels.[6] 2 patients who had previously been in cardiac failure developed it again while on levodopa, but 10 other patients with clinical or electrocardiographic evidence of heart disease showed no changes while on treatment.

Only 3 patients of the 21, or 14%, developed abnormal dyskinetic movements, and only 3 increased confusion. This contrasts with the commonly reported prevalence of dyskinesia of about 70%.[7,17] One important observation was that 5 patients became incontinent of urine at a time when their physical and mental state was improving; in all 5 the incontinence disappeared within a few weeks. Thus under these circumstances the development of incontinence should not be a reason for discontinuance of levodopa.

At the end of 6 months on levodopa, 12 patients were given orphenadrine 50 mg. three times daily in addition, because it has been suggested[8] that combined therapy gives better results than either drug alone. 7 of these 12 had an adverse reaction; 6 became confused and 1 developed the full picture of levodopa intoxication. None improved. All those who showed adverse reactions recovered completely when orphenadrine was withdrawn and levodopa continued in the same dose as before.

This trial thus shows that if levodopa is given to elderly patients with Parkinsonism in small doses with gradual increments, even the severely disabled patients so often encountered in geriatric practice can derive remarkable benefit. Perhaps what will strike geriatricians most is the discharge from continuing care of patients for whom this had previously been thought impossible.

These findings have been confirmed in all essentials by further personal experience of an additional 42 patients treated along the lines indicated by the trial. There were 25 men and 17 women, aged 58 to 86, with 28 aged 70 or more. The initial dose of levodopa was somewhat smaller than in the trial, being from 125 mg. once to three times daily. The increments have been of the same order, 125 mg. every 3 to 7 days, but the final dose averaged 1.5G rather than 2G per day. Again anticholinergic drugs have been withdrawn gradually, and only reintroduced in an attempt to control gross salivation or tremor. The most important single conclusion from the study of these patients is shown in Table 4. This is the relationship between initial mental state and degree of benefit. Of 23 patients in whom intellectual impairment was judged, on clinical and simple psychometric grounds, to be slight or absent, 17 have shown definite and worthwhile benefit from levodopa, 2 slight and doubtful benefit, and 4 no benefit. Of these 4, 2 are known or strongly suspected, of not taking their tablets, and using their disability to manipulate the home situation. Of 12 patients with moderate intellectual impairment, 5 have shown definite, 2 slight and 5 no benefit. None of the 7 with severe intellectual impairment have shown any benefit, and 2 died within the first few weeks. In this last group, the main side-effects of levodopa has been drowsiness, coming on within a few days of initiation of treatment, on doses as small as 125 mg. per day.

The frequency of side-effects has, as in the trial, been relatively low. Nausea and vomiting have been a rare problem, usually in the first week of treatment, and always disappearing with a pause in dose increments. Again, only 14% have had abnormal movements, despite a careful watch being kept, especially for the characteristic facial dyskinesia. Postural hypotension has been a problem in a small number of patients, particularly those given diuretics for oedema. A modest reduction in dose has always been sufficient to abolish it.

In patients with clear clinical evidence of severe heart disease, such as cardiomegaly or gallup rhythm, the increased mobility given by levodopa has on occasions led to the development of cardiac failure. This can be looked on as an unfortunate

Table 4

Relationship between initial mental
state and benefit from levodopa

Intellectual Impairment	Benefit from Levodopa Definite	Slight	None	Total
None or slight	17	2	4	23
Moderate	5	2	5	12
Severe	0	0	7	7

consequence of the benefits of treatment, and can be guarded against by common-sense precautions. Despite a high frequency of heart disease in these patients, the suggested need for continuous E.C.G. monitoring[9] has not been apparent.

A further consequence of increased mobility has been the occurrence of fractured femur in 2 patients (and 1 other not included in the present series). Increased mobility has not been accompanied by adequate safety in walking.

There is thus no doubt that levodopa used in the ways indicated can greatly benefit a substantial proportion of elderly patients with Parkinsonism, at an entirely acceptable risk of side effects. It is doubtful whether patients with severe intellectual impairment should be treated, but it is often difficult to deny the remote possibility of benefit from what is undoubtedly the patient's last hope.

The place of amantadine is much less certain. Its advantages are the speed with which its maximum effects are obtained, definite change being observable within a week, and its lower frequency of side-effects. But its maximum effectiveness is clearly much less than that of levodopa at its best. Some physicians use it as the first line of treatment for the elderly, and add levodopa if the benefits of amantadine are less than the patient's functional state requires; such a policy can lead to complex treatment regimes. Others use amantadine for two groups of patients: those who have minor disability from Parkinsonism, not thought sufficient to warrant levodopa,[14] and those in whom levodopa has failed or had to be abandoned. This is my own present policy, but as confidence with levodopa increases, at least the former group of patients becomes smaller, and the disadvantages of a policy that is neither entirely rational nor satisfactory become less.

References

1. Isaacs, B. and Akhtar, A.J. (1972). The set test: A rapid test of mental function in old people. Age and Ageing, 1, 222.

2. Boshes, B., Blonsky, E.R., Arbit, J. and Klein, K. (1969). Effect of L-Dopa on individual symptoms of Parkinsonism. Trans. Amer. Neurol. Ass., 94, 229.

3. Broe, G.A., Akhtar, A.J., Andrews, G.R. and Caird, F.I. (1972). Unpublished observations.

4. Broe, G.A. and Caird, F.I. (1973). Levodopa for Parkinsonism in elderly and demented patients. Med. J. Aust. 1, 630.

5. Brewis, M., Poskanzer, D.C., Rolland, C. and Miller, H. (1966). Neurological disease in an English city. Acta Neurol. Scand., 42, Suppl. 24.

6. Calne, D.B., Brennan, J., Spiers, A.S.D. and Stern, G.M. (1970). Hypotension caused by L-Dopa. Brit. Med. J., 1, 474.

7. Hughes, R.C., Polgar, J.G., Weightman, D. and Walton, J.N. (1971). L-Dopa in Parkinsonism and the influence of previous thalamotomy. Brit. Med. J. 1, 7.

8. Hughes, R.C., Polgar, J.G., Weightman, D. and Walton, J.N. (1971). Levodopa in Parkinsonism : The effects of withdrawal of anticholinergic drugs. Brit. Med. J., 2, 487.

9. Hunter, K.R., Hollman, A., Laurence, D.R. and Stern, G.M. (1971). Levodopa in Parkinsonian patients with heart disease. Lancet, 1, 932.

10. Jenkins, R.B. and Groh, R.H. (1970). Mental symptoms in Parkinsonian patients treated with L-Dopa. Lancet, 2, 177.

11. Kurland, L.T. (1958). In: Pathogenesis and treatment of Parkinsonism. p. 5. Fields, W.S. Ed. Springfield,

12. Marsh, G.G., Markham, C.M. and Ansel, R. (1971). Levodopa's awakening effect on patients with Parkinsonism. J. Neurol. Neurosurg. Psychiat., 34, 209.

13. Pallis, C.A. (1971). Parkinsonism : natural history and clinical features. Brit. Med. J., 3, 683.

14 Parker, J.D., Baxter, R.C.H., Curzon, G., Knill-Jones, R.P., Knott, P.J., Marsden, C.J., Tattersall, R. and Vollum, D. (1971). Treatment of Parkinson's disease with amantadine and levodopa. Lancet, 1, 1083.

15 Robinson, R.A. (1971). Assessment scales in a psychogeriatric unit. In: Assessment in cerebrovascular insufficiency. Stocker, G., Kuhn, R.A., Hall, P., Becker, G. and van der Veen, E., eds. Georg Thiene, Stuttgart, p. 89.

16 Sacks, O.W., Messeloff, C., Schartz, W., Goldfarb, A. and Kohl, M. (1970). Effects of l-dopa in patients with dementia. Lancet, 1, 1231 (letter).

17 Yahr, M.D., Duvoisin, R.C., Schear, M.J., Barrett, R.E. and Hoehn, M.M. (1969). Treatment of Parkinsonism with leveodopa. Arch. Neurol., 21, 343.

ADVANCES IN THE TREATMENT OF LEUKAEMIA

IRIS I.J.M. GIBSON

Consultant Physician
Southern General Hospital, Glasgow

The advances in the treatment of leukaemia are amongst the most
exciting in modern haematology, and discussion of these is very
relevant to medicine in old age, since every country which com-
piles statistics of mortality from leukaemia, except Japan,
shows a predominant rise in old people. There has, however, been
a great increase in the investigation of ill old people and in
the provision of laboratory facilities for this. Sternal marrow
aspiration is a minor procedure, and the indications for this
are unchanged by age. In addition, antibiotics and blood product
transfusion have allowed the survival of patients until accurate
diagnosis can be made. Increasing scientific accuracy suggests
that there has not been an actual rise in the numbers of old
people suffering from leukaemia but in the numbers actually
found to have leukaemia.

The majority of patients dying from leukaemia are beyond
middle age. Analysis of leukaemia deaths in New Zealand from
1950-54 showed that 57% were over fifty years of age, that more
than 60% of all leukaemias were acute and that 46% of acute

leukaemia occurred over the age of fifty. Analysis in the United States of America for the year 1949 showed a similar percentage over fifty.[4,1]

If deaths from acute leukaemia are plotted there are two peaks in the curve; under five years of age and over sixty. Some of the elderly will, of course, be cases of blastic termination of chronic myeloid leukaemia. The maximum incidence of chronic myeloid is at fifty years. Chronic lymphatic leukaemia is a disease of the elderly, rising progressively with age.

Since the treatment of acute leukaemia in adults is based upon that in children it is easy to illustrate the basic principles by a short description of the treatment of acute leukaemia in children. This is predominantly lymphoblastic leukaemia which is relatively amenable to chemotherapy. With modern therapy a child with an initial W.B.C. count below 5,000/cu.mm. can achieve 3-5 years of relatively active life.

Childhood leukaemia is now considered in three phases - induction of remission, consolidation and maintenance. Remission must be obtained for survival, and this can be brought about by potent drugs in combination used early in the disease. Therapy is aimed at various phases of the mitotic cycle and synthesis of D.N.A., R.N.A., and protein in active cells. Some drugs synchronize the mitosis of cells into one phase, so that other drugs can destroy these. Some drugs recruit resting cells into the mitotic cycle, thus exposing these to other drugs. Arbitrary tests of remission (that blood, bone marrow and cerebrospinal fluid are normal and there are no abnormal signs) can be achieved in 90% of previously untreated cases with synergistic therapy, such as combination of vincristine, daunorubicin and prednisone. Each drug has great toxicity singly, but in combination much smaller doses give more effective treatment with less toxicity. Each drug attacks the leukaemic process in a different way. If this effective combination fails there is a number of drugs and combinations available. The problems of infection, haemorrhage and hyperuricaemia can be treated by platelet transfusion, antibiotics and granulocyte transfusion and allopurinol.

Consolidation is a prolonged period of further intensive therapy after remission. This is essential to prevent rapid relapse, and different drugs are used. Methotrexate, 6 Mercaptopurine, L-asparaginase and cyclophosphamide, singly or cyclically, and prednisone can be used. With prolonged survival there is a relatively high incidence of meningeal leukaemia. Leukaemic cells are also found in other tissues which are out of reach of the vascular and lymphatic systems. Intrathecal methotrexate or cytosine arabinoside and irradiation of the central nervous system are used. The induction drugs may be given at regular intervals throughout consolidation.

A state of maintenance is achieved, and repeated marrow biopsy warns of relapse. Immunotherapy, methotrexate and repeated combined chemotherapy may be used at this time.

Many specialised centres have achieved considerable success. This has encouraged attempts to treat myeloblastic leukaemia in adults in a similar way. This is much more difficult but with combined therapy one-half to two-thirds of those treated have achieved remission of several months. Age is an important factor and older patients do less well. Treatment must be radical and quick. This is well illustrated by the work of Rosenthal and Moloney.[6] They obtained complete remission of 55% with average survival of eleven months by the use of drugs given intravenously. 1.5 mg. of Vincristine was given on the first day, with three-day courses of 2 mg. per kilogram cytosine arabinoside and 1 mg. per kilogram Daunorubicin. If blasts cleared from the blood marrow aspiration was performed. If blasts remained in the blood the programme was repeated. The induction drugs given cyclically did not maintain control, but reinduction was successful. Cytosine arabinoside is probably the most important drug.

It inhibits D.N.A. synthesis and synchronizes cell cycles, so
that the schedule of administration markedly influences results.
Daunorubicin, an anthracycline antitumour antibiotic, is also
an effective remission drug. In 1970 Crowther et al.[2] obtained
62% remission with these two drugs together. Later Crowther
et al.[3] obtained 54% complete remission with intermittent five-
day courses of these two drugs. These two successful programmes
use the best drugs when used singly, which have different side
effects. Toxicity is practically confined to pancytopenia and
oral ulceration and infection. The drugs are used intravenously,
have a short induction period, lead to rapid fall in blasts, and
can be given with allopurinol.

Other induction drugs include the new anthracycline antibiotic adriamycin, thiopurine analogues 6 mercaptopurine and 6
thioguanine. The most interesting drug is L-asparaginase, an
enzyme which catalyses the hydrolysis of L-asparagine. Leukaemic
cells die without asparagine, so die when it is destroyed by the
anzyme. Normal cells do not. This drug exploits the biochemical
abnormality of leukaemic cells. However resistance develops
readily and Crowther and his colleagues did not find that the
addition of this drug improved results. Steroids are still
important drugs for the prevention of haemorrhage and promotion
of well being.

This is a brief description of therapy for guidance only.

Other drugs singly or cyclically are used for consolidation
- 6-mercaptopurine, cyclophosphamide, methotrexate, alternate
cytosine arabinoside and daunorubicin, alternate cytosine
arabinoside and thioguanine.

Methotrexate is useful in maintenance. Immunotherapy with
irradiated leukaemia cells and B.C.G. may prove useful.[3]

So far remission rates in acute myeloblastic leukaemia have
been worst with older patients. The choice of population for
clinical trials, however, has not been from patients in geriatric

wards and this may give a false idea of leukaemia in age. Trials in geriatric medicine are now needed, and treatment is within the scope of geriatric medicine, within specialised units.

There has been progress in the control of chronic myeloid leukaemia. The 1968 M.R.C.[5] trial showed that Busulphan was the most effective therapy in controlling the W.B.C. count, anaemia and spleen size and improving life. The drug is given orally, in a dose of 4-6 mg./day until W.B.C. count reaches 20,000/cu.mm. or platelet count 100,000/cu.mm. The drug is then stopped, but can be resumed in smaller dosage to control W.B.C. count at 10,000/cu.mm. Average survival is 3-4 years. If too much is given irreversible bone marrow aplasia is produced. If the drug is given for several years a wasting syndrome with pigmentation anorexia, and sometimes pulmonary fibrosis, may be produced. If resistance develops there are now a number of other oral drugs worth trying - hydroxyurea, pipobroman, piposulfan, dibromomannitol, uracil mustard and 6-mercaptopurine.

Chronic lymphatic leukaemia should only be treated if it affects the patient by anaemia, thrombocytopenia, haemolysis, large gland masses, weight loss or exhaustion. It is a disorder of the elderly which rarely becomes blastic, and may not interfere with the patient's life. Owing to impairment of antibody formation, haemolysis and infection are the greatest problems. Steroids alone will often control haemolysis, but if specific treatment is required chlorambucil in an initial dose of 0.1 - 0.2 mg./Kg. with reduction after approximately a month, is a satisfactory drug. Cyclophosphamide and local radiotherapy may be useful. Uracil mustard can be effective.[7]

It is obvious that geriatric medicine provides considerable opportunity for further research and that further advances can be made within the geriatric service by those with experience in treating the various forms of leukaemia.

References

1. Cooke, J.V. (1954). The occurrence of leukaemia. Blood, 9, 340.

2. Crowther, D., Bateman, C.J.T., Vartan, C.P., Whitehouse, J.M.A., Malpas, J.S., Fairley, G.H. and Bodley Scott, R. (1970). Combination chemotherapy using L-asparaginase, daunorubicin and cytosine arabinoside in adults with acute myelogenous leukaemia. Brit. Med. J., IV, 513.

3. Crowther, D., Powles, R.L., Bateman, C.J.T., Beard, M.E.J., Gauci, C.L., Wrigley, P.F.M., Malpas, J.S., Hamilton Fairley, A. and Bodley Scott, R. (1973). Management of adult acute myelogenous leukaemia. Brit. Med. J., I, 131.

4. Gunz, F.W. and Hough R.F. (1956). Acute leukaemia over the age of fifty. A study of its incidence and natural history. Blood, 11, 882.

5. Medical Research Council Report (1968). Brit. Med. J., I, 201.

6. Rosenthal, D.S. and Moloney, W.C. (1972). The treatment of acute granulocytic leukaemia in adults. New Eng. J. Med., 286, 1176.

7. Wilkinson, J.F., Bourne, M.D. and Israels, M.C.G. (1963). Treatment of leukaemias and reticulosis with uracil mustard. Brit. Med. J., I, 1563.

PROGRESS IN GERIATRIC GASTROENTEROLOGY

IAIN W. DYMOCK

Senior Lecturer in Medicine
University of Manchester

Introduction

In the past decade there has been significant progress in the management of patients with gastro-intestinal disorders. Significant advances have been made possible both by improved investigational techniques such as fibre-optic endoscopy and the use of radionucleides for organ-scanning and tests of intestinal absorption and by the introduction of new therapeutic agents.

Gastro-Intestinal Endoscopy

Following the original application of fibre-optics to endoscopy by Hirschowitz[12] in 1958 flexible gastroscopes and oesophagoscopes were developed which with progressive modification have provided the gastroenterologist with the capability of examining the oesophagus, stomach and duodenum under direct vision and at the same time obtain biopsies and samples for cytology from the optimum sites. In addition photographic facilities are available so that a permanent record can be obtained for teaching or other purposes. It is usual to premedicate the patient with atropine and diazepam and to apply local anaesthetic spray to the pharynx, so that the examination can be performed with the minimum of inconvenience in a fully conscious patient. There are few contraindications to this type of endoscopy and it has been used with success in both the young and the elderly. Recently I performed an oesophagoscopy on a ninety-three year old man with dysphagia in whom a barium swallow had revealed a lesion suggestive of malignancy. At endoscopy he had an obvious oesophagitis which was confirmed by biopsy and which has since responded to medical measures thus avoiding the general anaesthetic which would have been necessary for examination with the standard rigid instrument. In oesophageal disorders the main role of the fibre-endoscopes is in the investigation of dysphagia and the establishment of a diagnosis with biopsy confirmation in patients with lesions on a barium swallow.

The diagnosis of gastric carcinoma can be facilitated by endoscopy and the differentiation of benign from malignant gastric ulceration made possible thus permitting the benign lesions to be treated medically. Atrophic gastritis can be readily identified by the loss of mucosal folds and the ease with which the vascular pattern in the mucosa can be seen. Finally in patients who have upper alimentary symptoms with a negative barium x-ray or with occult alimentary blood loss the examination may reveal the responsible lesion.

More recently it has been possible to enter the duodenum with the identification of duodenal ulceration[20], duodenitis[2], and duodenal tumours.[3] A further development has been the use of the endoscope to identify and cannulate the ampulla of Vater in patients with obstructive jaundice and perform retrograde cholangiography. Using this technique Cotton and his colleagues[7] were able to obtain such radiographs in almost 70% of the patients they examined.

Similar instruments have been developed for the examination of the colon[9] and these colonoscopes can be passed along the entire length of the colon although it is more usual to be able to examine as far as the hepatic or splenic flexures. Certainly they can give good views of the colonic lumen in the "blind-area" of the sigmoid and the differentiation of carcinoma from diverticular disease in this area has proved possible.[8]

Gastric Ulceration

Gastric ulceration occurs frequently in the elderly, Mulsow[15] finding that 10% of all ulcers occurred in the over sixties, whilst one-third of all ulcer deaths were in this age group. Evidence of a similarly high mortality was recorded by McKeown[14] who found that in a series of 65 patients with proven gastric ulceration the ulcer had been the main cause of death in 34 of them. When these figures are considered it becomes obvious that gastric ulceration in the elderly should be looked upon as a serious condition requiring urgent treatment.

Most surgeons treat gastric ulceration by partial gastrectomy with a gastro-duodenal anastomosis. The results of this operation are good, the incidence of post-operative syndromes low and recurrence is infrequent. Nevertheless with the risk of such surgery particularly in older patients, physicians and surgeons have sought a means of treating these ulcers medically. Unfortunately antacids and anti-cholinergic drugs, whilst they may provide symptomatic relief, do not heal these ulcers. However, the liquorice derivatives, carbenoxolone sodium (Biogastonre) and deglycyrrhizinized liquorice can effect healing in the ambulant patient.[10,21,22] Unfortunately carbenoxolone sodium may produce side effects particularly in older people[22] with hypertension, oedema and hypokalaemia. Fortunately deglycyrrhizinized liquorice is free from these complications and is at present the treatment of choice. Failure of a gastric ulcer to heal within six weeks should raise the possibility of malignancy and these patients should be considered candidates for surgery then.

Duodenal Diverticula

Diverticula of the duodenum were once regarded as a clinical rarity but recent reports have emphasised both their frequent occurrence and the high incidence of associated complications. Bockus[4] has estimated that they occur in 10% of people over the age of 55 years and that the incidence subsequently increases as years advance. Recently Clark[5] has described fifteen patients with either single or multiple diverticula who had a variety of associated disease states. In 8 of his patients the diverticulae were multiple. The principle symptoms were diarrhoea (5 patients), iron deficiency anaemia (5 patients), dyspepsia (3 patients), weight loss (3 patients) and anorexia (3 patients). Two patients presented with osteomalacia. Further examination and investigation revealed that no less than 10 of the 15 patients had anaemia and the causation included folate, iron and vitamin B12 deficiency. Intestinal malabsorption was common and both this and the vitamin deficiency states were attributed to intestinal bacterial colonisation with bile-salt deconjugation.[11]

These reports are of particular interest and suggest that in elderly patients with malabsorption syndromes or vitamin deficiency states an organic lesion such as a duodenal or jejunal diverticulum should be considered as a primary cause. These patients respond well to antibiotic therapy, such as the tetracyclines or lincomycin and surgical management is rarely necessary.

The Malabsorption Syndrome in the Elderly

The classical presenting symptoms in the malabsorption syndrome of weight loss, diarrhoea, anaemia and vitamin deficiency will occur frequently in old people and only rarely are they due to intestinal malabsorption. However recent work suggests that minor degrees of intestinal malabsorption occur frequently in old people[24] with associated mucosal structural changes.[23] In this age group patients have been described with classical coeliac disease[1,19] but in most instances this is not of the gluten sensitive type but is rather associated with another intestinal pathology such as duodenal diverticula[5] or intestinal ischaemia[13] or intestinal colonisation producing a malabsorption syndrome due to bile salt deconjugation.

The assessment of intestinal function in the elderly is made difficult by the need to perform a variety of tests. Most of these require good hepatic or renal function which is often impaired in the elderly and both stool and urine collections may be difficult. No single test is adequate but a balanced assessment from the measurement of a serum folate, vitamin B12 absorption, stool fat excretion and urinary indican output should be of value. Only rarely will the clinician consider a jejunal biopsy but a barium follow-through examination is both more acceptable and more likely to succeed.

Diverticular Disease of the Colon

Diverticular disease of the colon appears to be a disease of Western civilisation.[17] It may present a wide spectrum of clinical features ranging from the completely asymptomatic individual to those with peritonitis or pericolic abscess. The incidence of this condition appears to be increasing in the United Kingdom[6] particularly in females. The incidence also appears to increase with age[16] and reaches 60% in female patients over the age of 80.

The aetiology, however, remains obscure and although there is good evidence that there is a neuromuscular inco-ordination in the colon[18] and that obesity, constipation and a low-roughage diet may be implicated, no single factor has been identified.

In patients who present with a pericolic abscess or peritonitis the management is surgical but in the majority the symptoms are constipation, occasional diarrhoea and pre-defaecation hypogastric colic. Fortunately these respond readily to a high-residue diet or methyl-cellulose and an antispasmodic such as mebeverine. More drastic measures are rarely required.

References

1 Badenoch, J. (1960). Brit. med. J., 2, 880.
2 Belber, J.P. (1969). Gastroint. Endoscopy, 15, 160.
3 Belber, J.P. (1970). IInd World Congress of Gastrointest. Endoscopy.
4 Bockus, H.L. (1966). Gastroenterology. p. 128. Saunders, Philadelphia.
5 Clark, A.N.G. (1972). Age and Ageing, 1, 14.
6 Cleave, T.L., Campbell, G.B. and Painter, N.S. (1969). Diabetes, Coronary Thrombosis and the Saccharine Disease. Wright, Bristol.
7 Cotton, P.B., Salmon, P.R., Blumgart, L.H., Burwood, R.J., Davies, G.T., Lawrie, B.W., Pierce, J.W. and Read, A.E. (1972). Lancet, 1, 53.
8 Dean, A.C.B. and Newell, J.P. (1973). Brit. J. Surg., 60, 633.
9 Dean, A.C.B. and Shearman, D.J.C. (1970). Lancet, 1, 550.
10 Doll, R., Hill, I.D., Hutton, C.F. and Underwood, D.J.H. (1962). Lancet, 2, 793.
11 Gorbach, S.L. and Tabaqchali, S. (1969). Gut, 10, 936.
12 Hirschowitz, B.I., Curtis, L.E. and Peters, C.W. (1958). Gastroenterology, 35, 50.
13 Kennedy Watt, J., Watson, W.C. and Haase, S. (1967). Brit. med. J., 2, 199.
14 McKeown, F. (1965). Pathology of the Aged, p. 134, Butterworths, London.
15 Mulsow, F.W. (1941). Amer. J. Dig. Dis., 8, 112.
16 Painter, N.S. (1964). Ann. Roy. Coll. Surgeons of England, 34, 98.
17 Painter, N.S. and Burkitt, D.P. (1971). Brit. med. J., 2, 450.
18 Painter, N.S., Truelove, S.C., Ardran, G.M. and Tuckey, M. (1965). Gastroenterology, 49, 165.

19. Ryder, J.B. (1963). Geront. Clin., 5, 30.
20. Shearman, D.J.C., Warwick, R.R.G., MacLeod, I.B. and Dean, A.C.B. (1971). Lancet, 1, 726.
21. Turpie, A.G.G., Runcie, J. and Thomson, T.J. (1969). Gut, 10, 299.
22. Turpie, A.G.G. and Thomson, T.J. (1965). Gut, 6, 591.
23. Webster, S.G.P. (1973). Personal communication.
24. Webster, S.G.P. and Leeming, J.T. (1973). In preparation.

RECENT ADVANCES IN RESPIRATORY DISEASES

ANWAR J. AKHTAR

Consultant Physician in Geriatric Medicine,
Eastern General Hospital, Edinburgh

Ventilatory Capacity

The ventilatory capacity of elderly patients is frequently measured in hospital wards, out-patient clinics and as part of research projects. This is usually done by measuring the forced expiratory volume in one second (FEV_1) and the forced vital capacity (FVC). In spite of the extensive use of these tests in the elderly, very little data is available about values in the general elderly population. There is no shortage of data for young and middle-aged subjects,[3,8,14] and until recently predicted normal values for the elderly were arrived at by extrapolation. Milne and Williamson[21] in Edinburgh measured the ventilatory capacity of 215 men and 272 women, aged between 62 and 90 years, who formed a random sample of 27,000 older people living in a defined area of the city. A vitalograph sirometer was used to determine the FEV_1 and FVC. They found that the decrease of the FEV_1 with age was not significant in men, but was significant in women at the 1% level. The decrease in the FVC was significant at the 5% level in men and 1% level in women. Predicted values for normal men and women for the FEV_1 are given in Figure 1, and for the FVC in Figure 2. The respiratory function variable is shown on the ordinate and height (mm.) on the abscissa with lines to allow prediction of normal values at four different ages. Milne and Williamson also compared the multiple regression equations based on the mean of three and the best of three readings for the FEV_1 and FVC. They found that the regression lines for the mean of three readings and the best of three readings could be considered parallel. The difference in the intercept values were of the order of 100 ml. or less, and therefore the difference between mean of three and best of three readings is not of clinical importance. The FEV_1 calculated from some of the regression equations in the literature for a man aged 70 years and 1.6 m. tall range from 2.21 L[8] to 2.41 L[3] and from 1.59 L to 1.74 L for a woman aged 70 years, 1.5 m. tall. The corresponding values derived from the regression equations of Milne and Williamson were 1.96 L and 1.46 L. Values for FVC are similarly exaggerated in the literature.

These values clearly demonstrate the importance of using regression equations based on a sample of the elderly population for the prediction of the FEV_1 and the FVC of older people.

Distribution of Pulmonary Ventilation and Perfusion

Holland et al.[16] investigated the distribution of ventilation and perfusion of six normal subjects aged between 65 and 75 years by studies with radioactive xenon. They found that by comparison with normal young men; (a) the blood flow to the upper zones increased although it still remained greater in the lower zones; (b) ventilation distribution during a vital capacity inspiration was similar to that seen in younger subjects, and (c) in five of the six the distribution of ventilation in the resting, tidal volume range was not preferential to the lower zones as it was in young men. This was probably caused

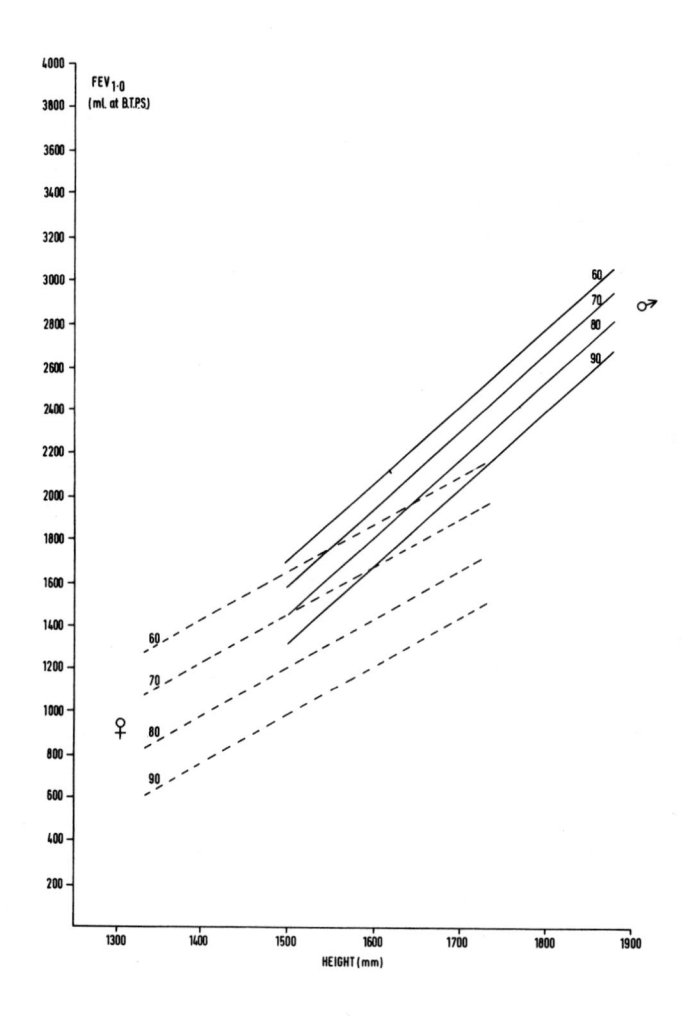

Figure 1

Reproduced by kind permission of the authors, and the editor of Clinical Science.[21]

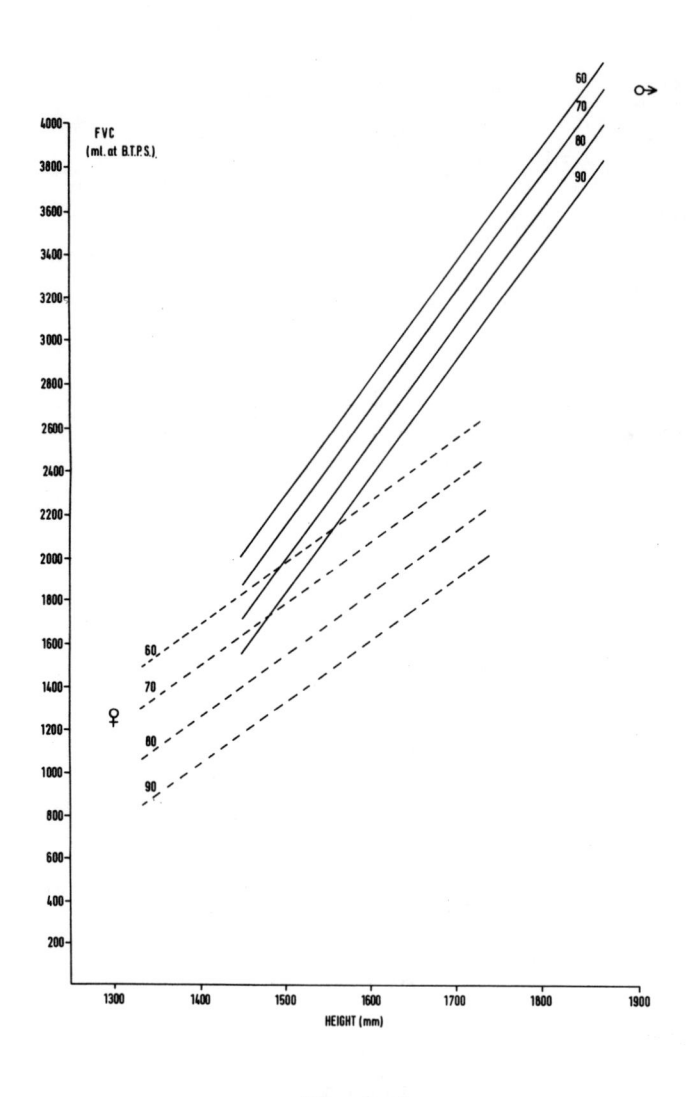

Figure 2

Reproduced by kind permission of the authors, and the editor of Clinical Science.[21]

by airways closure in the lower lung zones. These findings suggest that in the elderly subject there is a significant regional ventilation perfusion impairment during quiet breathing which may explain in part the reported increase in alveolar arterial oxygen difference with advancing age.[20,23]

The Regression of Respiratory and Cardiac Function with Increasing Age

Ericsson and Irnell[12] measured lung volumes and physical work capacity in healthy individuals between the ages of 57 and 71 years. There were 20 subjects between the ages of 67 and 71. Work capacity was measured by using a bicycle ergometer. The work load was increased in steps of 200 and 300 Kpm/min. and each period lasted six minutes until a heart rate of 170/minute was reached. No significant correlation was found between lung volumes and physical work capacity or between ventilatory capacity and physical work capacity. These experiments were repeated five years later on the same subjects.[13] It was found that the regression of ventilatory capacity was not as great over five years as the regression of work capacity. They did, however, find a significant correlation between workload at a given pulse rate and age. It seems possible that the regression of physiological function with increasing age may have different time courses for the respiratory and circulatory systems.

Chronic Respiratory Disease in the Elderly Population

Caird and Akhtar[6] studied a random sample of 83 men and 217 women aged 65 and over, living in their own homes in northern Glasgow. A full medical history including the Medical Research Council standard questionnaire on respiratory symptoms,[17] and a detailed clinical examination was carried out, except in those whose general condition necessitated examination at home rather than at a clinic. A six foot postero-anterior and left lateral radiograph was taken and the FEV_1 and FVC were measured. Chest radiographs were obtained in 277 subjects (92% of the total), and they were classified on the basis of the radiologist's report as being normal, or as showing either minor or significant abnormality. Examples of minor abnormality were pleural thickening, a primary tuberculous complex or a small focus of healed post primary tuberculosis, which were not thought to give rise to abnormality of respiratory function, nor to require further follow-up. Significant abnormalities included pulmonary tuberculosis with more substantial lesions, often with fibrotic contracture of one or both upper lobes, bronchial carcinoma, industrial lung disease and miscellaneous abnormalities such as fibrotic lesions not typical of any specific respiratory disorder. Chronic bronchitis was diagnosed clinically by means of the M.R.C. questionnaire on respiratory symptoms. No significant respiratory disease was considered present in 58% of the men and 80% of the women. Nineteen of 48 men (38%) and 28 of 156 women (18%) without significant respiratory disease had minor radiological abnormalities. The prevalence of chronic bronchitis was found to be 26% in men and 13% in women, and did not vary with age. An impressive increase in the prevalence of chronic bronchitis with declining socio-economic status was found in men, but not in women. In both sexes current smoking habits were related to the prevalence of chronic bronchitis. It was 12% in those who had never smoked and approached 50% in those who smoked more than 15 cigarettes a day. Other respiratory diseases found included asthma (2% women), pulmonary tuberculosis (9% of men and 4% of women), and industrial lung disease (4% of men), but chronic bronchitis was quantitatively the most important chronic respiratory disorder encountered. The overall prevalence of chronic respiratory disease in the elderly was 40% in men and 20% in women.

Bronchial Carcinoma

Bronchial carcinoma rivals chronic bronchitis as an important cause of morbidity and mortality in the elderly. It accounts for approximately 7% of male and 2% of female deaths over the age of 65 in the Registrar General for Scotland 1971 figures.[24] In England and Wales the peak mortality in males was found to be between the ages of 70 and 75 in 1963.[9] Surgery in selected cases has generally been regarded as the only radical means of treatment offering any hope of a permanent cure. In the elderly this poses problems of its own. Belcher and Anderson[2] analysed the results of surgical treatment of bronchial carcinoma in 50 patients over the age of 70 years. They found an operative mortality following pneumonectomy of 33%. The overall two year survival was 12% and no patient survived five years. These investigators questioned the wisdom of surgical treatment of bronchial carcinoma in patients over the age of 70. Bates[1] reported the results of surgery for bronchial carcinoma in 100 patients over the age of 70 treated between 1950 and 1968, in the North Middlesex Hospital, London. 89 patients had resections and 12 were inoperable at thoracotomy. The operative mortality with pneumonectomy was 24% and 14% with lobectomy. Only three patients were alive 10 years after surgery.

It would seem from these findings that lung resection in the elderly is an extremely hazardous procedure and should only be undertaken in carefully selected patients.

The findings of the Medical Research Council trial[18] throw serious doubt on the role of surgery in the treatment of oat-cell carcinoma, as radiotherapy was shown to be marginally better than surgery. Only clinically operable cases were admitted to the trial. Radiotherapy is therefore the treatment of choice for oat-cell tumours in the elderly.

The small rounded peripheral opacity measuring about 1-4 cm. on the chest radiograph of an elderly patient can present serious problems. Is it tuberculosis or is it tumour? A previous chest X-ray, tomography and the tuberculin test may confirm the diagnosis but in a high proportion of cases the aetiology remains a mystery. Dr. G.K. Crompton in Edinburgh[10] treats elderly patients with such lesions on the chest radiographs with a single "test" dose of radiotherapy sufficient to produce shrinkage of a carcinoma but insufficient to upset the patient. He is of the view that this should not be done under anti-tuberculosis chemotherapy cover. Should the lesion remain the same size or enlarge after radiotherapy, treatment with anti-tuberculosis chemotherapy is then commenced, but if shrinkage occurs further radiotherapy is given. It is hoped that radiotherapy used in this way will reduce the need for surgical treatment in the old, and cut down the number of patients who are treated with anti-tuberculosis drugs until the malignant nature of the small peripheral lesion becomes obvious, at which stage the disease is often so far advanced that no form of curative therapy can be considered.

Bronchial Asthma

Bronchial asthma may be chronic or episodic. Episodic asthma presents few diagnostic problems but chronic bronchial asthma, especially in the elderly, is not infrequently mistaken for chronic bronchitis. The patient may therefore be denied the benefits of modern treatment which may transform him from living as a housebound respiratory cripple to leading a normal active existence. Corticosteroids have revolutionised the outlook of the chronic asthmatic. They remain the most important advance in the treatment of bronchial asthma. Walsh and Grant[26] analysed the results of treatment in 245 adult chronic asthmatics. 33 patients were over the age of 60 years but were not analysed separately. These patients were selected for long-term corticosteroid treatment with careful clinical assessment of the severity of symptoms, both historical and when the patient was seen, and detailed enquiry into whether measures other than corticosteroids had been used to full advantage. The patient was initially given inert tablets identical in appearance and taste with 5 mg. prednisolone tablets. The FEV_1 was recorded daily. This was to establish a base line of FEV_1 readings. As soon as stable base line readings had been established, 5 mg. prednisolone tablets were substituted for the inert tablets without the patient's knowledge. The FEV_1 was recorded for a further seven days and the patient's response was assessed as the percentage increase in the FEV_1 during corticosteroid treatment. On the basis of the pattern of response, the appropriate treatment regimen was selected. The treatment regimens varied from daily prednisolone of 10 mg. a day to thrice weekly prednisolone on three consecutive days in a dose of 20 mg. a day. The great majority of patients improved dramatically on prednisolone and were able to live a normal life. The incidence of fractures occurring either spontaneously or as a result of minor trauma was much higher in patients on continuous treatment (15%) than in those on intermittent treatment (1%). Wedge fractures of vertebral bodies and cough fractures of ribs accounted for all but one of the incidents. Intermittent corticosteroid treatment would appear to be the treatment of choice in the elderly whenever possible.

Disodium cromoglycate (Intal) has been used extensively in young asthmatics and has been found to have a beneficial effect in a significant proportion of patients. Grant[15] however has reservations about the value of this drug because of the reliance on subjective criteria by many of the investigators assessing this substance rather than on objective tests of pulmonary function. The role of disodium cromoglycate has yet to be established in the elderly asthmatic.

Beclomethasone dipropionate is the first effective steroid aerosol for the treatment of bronchial asthma which does not appear to have significant systemic effects when small doses are inhaled. Brown et al.[4] used beclomethasone dipropionate in aerosol form for the treatment of 60 cases of chronic bronchial astham. 37 patients were already on oral steroids and 28 of these were successfully transferred to the aerosol and no biochemical evidence of adrenal suppression was found. Only 4 patients were over the age of 60. Of these 3 responded successfully to the aerosol. Clark[7] studied the effect of beclomethasone dipropionate on 17 patients with asthma. 8 of these were transferred from prednisolone to the new treatment. The steroid aerosol seemed to exert a topical corticosteroid action on the airways with a satisfactory therapeutic result. 5 of the 17 patients treated were 60 years of age or over. The dose of beclomethasone dipropionate ranged from 100 ug. four times daily to 200 ug. four times daily. The mode of action of this substance is not fully understood but it seems from the small amount of evidence available that beclomethasone dipropionate does have a local topical effect on the bronchi. The role of this substance needs to be further clarified but if the findings of preliminary investigations are confirmed by more extensive trials, beclomethasone dipropionate will have an important place in the management of the elderly asthmatic.

Tuberculosis

The importance of cryptic disseminated tuberculosis has been appreciated for some years but Proudfoot et al[22] emphasised its importance in the elderly. They reviewed the case records of 40 adults in Edinburgh in whom the diagnosis of disseminated tuberculosis was made between 1954 and 1967. 24 patients had overt disseminated tuberculosis with evidence of the disease on the chest radiograph and 16 had cryptic disease with initially normal chest radiographs. The peak age incidence of disseminated tuberculosis in this series was in the eighth decade, and 58% of the patients were over the age of 60 years. They emphasise the importance of suspecting cryptic disseminated tuberculosis in all elderly patients presenting with a pyrexia of unknown origin. In a proportion of these patients a bacteriological diagnosis is possible and may be achieved by sputum examination, liver biopsy, marrow biopsy and in some cases cerebro-spinal fluid examination. If extensive investigation proves unhelpful, the patient should be given the benefit of a therapeutic trial with anti-tuberculosis chemotherapy. The drugs chosen must be effective against the tubercle bacillus only and streptomycin is therefore not used. Proudfoot et al. recommended P.A.S. and isoniazid but ethambutol can now be added or used in combination with isoniazid to replace the relatively toxic drug P.A.S. The criteria used to assess the effectiveness of the therapeutic trial are of paramount importance. These are a fall in the temperature within a week of starting treatment, improved well-being within two to six weeks, gain in weight, and in anaemic patients, a rise in haemoglobin.

For many years now P.A.S., isoniazid and streptomycin have been the first line drugs for the treatment of tuberculosis. In recent years several new preparations effective against the tubercle bacillus have been developed. Not all have proved viable alternatives to traditional chemotherapy but ethambutol and rifampicin are certainly threatening the pre-eminence of P.A.S. and streptomycin as drugs of first choice in the treatment of tuberculosis in the elderly. Ethambutol is highly effective and is already replacing P.A.S. in some centres in this country. It is particularly useful in the elderly because of its relative freedom from toxicity compared with the gastro-intestinal side effects of P.A.S. and the vestibular damage associated with treatment with streptomycin. Retrobulbar neuritis, which is rare, seems to be its only serious side effect.[11] It is given in a dose of 20 mg. per kilogram of body weight per day. Rifampicin is a derivative of rifamycin which is administered orally. It is virtually free of toxicity when given daily and is given in a single daily dose before breakfast of 450 mg. In a controlled clinical trial of four six-month regimens of anti-tuberculosis chemotherapy supervised by the Medical Research Council[19] in East Africa, it was found that streptomycin, isoniazid and rifampicin given daily for six months was highly effective in the treatment of extensive pulmonary tuberculosis. It seems likely that regimens containing rifampicin may reduce the total duration of treatment for anything other than extensive tuberculous disease from the current minimum of 18 months to even six months. The British Thoracic and Tuberculosis Association is shortly to conduct trials in which patients will be treated for between six months and eighteen months, and will be given rifampicin, isoniazid and streptomycin if they are under 60 and ethambutol in place of streptomycin if they are over 60.[5] It seems possible that combinations of rifampicin, ethambutol and isoniazid will become the treatment of choice for the elderly patient. The duration of treatment of tuberculosis is also likely to be dramatically reduced because of the advent of these new drugs.

References

1. Bates, M. (1970). Results of surgery for bronchial carcinoma in patients aged 70 and over. Thorax, 25, 77.
2. Belcher, J.R. and Anderson, R. (1965). Surgical treatment of carcinoma of the bronchus. Brit. Med. J., 1, 948.
3. Berglund, E., Birath, G., Bjure, J., Grimby, G., Kjellmer, I., Sandgrist, L. and Soddrholm, B. (1963). Spirometric studies in normal subjects. 1. Forced spirograms in subjects between 7 and 70 years of age. Acta Medica Scandinavica., 173, 185.
4. Brown, H.M., Storey, G. and George, W.H.S. (1972). Beclomethasone dipropionate: A new steroid aerosol for the treatment of allergic asthma. Brit. Med. J., 1, 585.
5. Campbell, I. Personal Communication.
6. Caird, F.I. and Akhtar, A.J. (1972). Chronic respiratory disease in the elderly: A population study. Thorax, 27, 764.
7. Clark, P.J.H. (1972). Effect of beclomethasone dipropionate delivered by aerosol in patients with asthma. Lancet 1, 1361.
8. Cotes, J.E. (1968). Lung function. Blackwell Scientific Publications, Oxford.
9. Crofton, J. and Douglas, A. (1969). Respiratory diseases. Blackwell Scientific Publications Limited.
10. Crompton, G.K. Personal Communication.
11. Elibold, J.E. (1966). The ocular toxicity of ethambutol and its relation to dose. Ann. N.Y. Acad. Sci., 135, 904.
12. Ericsson, P. and Irnell, L. (1969). Physical work capacity and static lung volumes in elderly people. Acta. Medica. Scandinavica, 185, 185.
13. Ericsson, P. and Irnell, L. (1969). Effect of five years ageing on ventilatory capacity and physical work capacity in elderly people. Acta. Medica. Scandinavica, 185, 193.
14. Ferris, B.G., Anderson, D.O. and Zick Mantel, R. (1965). Prediction values for screening tests of pulmonary function. American Review of Respiratory Diseases, 91, 252.

15 Grant, I.W.B. (1971). The treatment of bronchial asthma. British Tuberculosis and Thoracic Association Review, 1, 43.

16 Holland, J., Milic-Emili, J., Macklem, P.T. and Bates, D.V. (1968). Regional distribution of pulmonary ventilation and perfusion in elderly subjects. J. Clin. Invest., 47, 81.

17 Medical Research Council (1966). Questionnaire on Respiratory Symptoms.

18 Medical Research Council (1966). Comparative trial of surgery and radiotherapy for the primary treatment of small celled or oat celled carcinoma of the bronchus. Lancet, 2, 979.

19 Medical Research Council (1972). Controlled clinical trial of short course (six months) regimes of chemotherapy for treatment of pulmonary tuberculosis. Lancet 1, 1079.

20 Mellemgarrd, K. (1966). The alveolar - arterial oxygen difference: its size and components in normal man. Acta. Physiol. Scandinavica, 67, 10.

21 Milne, J.S. and Williamson, J. (1972). Respiratory function tests in older people. Clin. Sci., 42, 371.

22 Proudfoot, A.P., Akhtar, A.J., Douglas, A.C. and Horne, N.W. (1969). Miliary tuberculosis in adults. Brit. Med. J., 2, 273.

23 Raine, J.N. and Bishop, J.M. (1963). A - a difference in oxygen tension and physiological dead space in normal man. J. App. Physiol., 18, 284.

24 Registrar General for Scotland (1971). Annual Report of the Registrar General for Scotland (1969). Part I: Mortality Statistics. H.M.S.O., Edinburgh.

25 Smith, N.J. and Tevey, G.F. (1968). Clinical trial of disodium cromglycate in treatment of asthma in children. Brit. Med. J., 2, 340.

26 Walsh, D.S. and Grant, I.W.B. (1966). Cortical steroids in treatment of chronic asthma. Brit. Med. J., 2, 796.

RECENT ADVANCES IN CARDIOLOGY

ROBIN D. KENNEDY

Consultant Geriatrician
Stobhill Hospital, Glasgow

Cardiac disease is one of the commonest causes of morbidity and
mortality in the elderly. In Scotland 37% of all old people,
that is, those aged 65 or more, die of heart disease, be they
male or female. Furthermore, the death rate from cardiac disease
accelerates rapidly with age in both sexes. In women, it doubles
in each decade from 65 years upwards.[9] According to the returns
of the Registrar General for Scotland, the majority of these
deaths are thought to be due to ischaemic heart disease. A
smaller number of deaths are certified as being due to hypertensive heart disease or rheumatic heart disease. There is also
a large group of people who die from other forms of heart disease, often with rather unsatisfactory diagnoses such as
myocardial insufficiency, or senile cardiac failure.

It is no longer justified to accept that heart disease in
the elderly is synonymous with ischaemic heart disease. Increasing interest in the pathology of the aged has shown that many old
people are subject to cardiac conditions which can be present at

any age. Again, several conditions occur affecting the cardiac system in the elderly which are almost exclusive to the older person.

Degenerative calcific valve disease is one of the commonest pathological abnormalities noted in the elderly. It has been found in up to 37% of subjects over 75 years of age when submitted to postmortem. Generally it takes the form of calcific nodules in the aortic valve cusps, occurring at the base of these cusps. Apart from producing the typical murmur of aortic sclerosis, such deposits are generally of no significance, though occasionally they can be the site of endocarditis.

However, about 6% of the elderly have actual aortic valve stenosis, and the cause of such stenosis has been in dispute for many years. Congenital, rheumatic, or ageing processes have all been incriminated as aetiological factors, but it seems likely that any of these processes may be responsible for the valve deformity, and that such deformity can often be correlated to the age of the person.

Pomerance[8] has recently confirmed that three definite pathological varieties of aortic valve stenosis in the elderly exist. The most frequent cause in the 65-74 year old group was found by her to be calcification of congenital bicuspid aortic valves. Over the age of 75 degenerative calcification was the main cause of isolated aortic stenosis; and in the very elderly was the sole finding in the stenosed aortic valve. Though forming the smallest group, inflammatory valve disease occurred at all ages, though much more frequently in those of younger years. There were a very few instances of inflammatory changes occurring on congenitally bicuspid valves, and again this was seen in the younger subject.

In the mitral valve rheumatic heart disease is known to occur in about 4% of the elderly.[1] Such a diseased valve is subject to the usual complications which occur in younger individuals. A further condition affecting the mitral valve, mainly in the elderly, is degenerative calcification. This occurs in the mitral ring and not the cusps proper. It increases in incidence with advancing age, and is about three times commoner in women than in men.[7] Often the only clinical evidence of its presence is an apical systolic murmur due to the distortion of the posterior valve cusp, causing incompetence. This calcification generally starts near the attachment of the cusps to the interventricular septum. This is near the bundle of His. and its main branches. Incomplete heart block may, therefore, accompany such calcification and a further complication may ensue if calcium ulcerates through the valve cusps, forming a possible site for endocarditis. The cause or causes of such mitral ring calcification are not yet clear.

Cardiac amyloidosis occurs with increasing frequency in the elderly person. This form of primary amyloid disease is entirely localised to the heart. Pomerance[6] estimates that at least 10% of patients over the age of 80, and 50% of those over 90 show myocardial amyloid deposits at autopsy. Clinically in many of her subjects cardiac failure was present, often with no detectable aetiology. One interesting feature in people with retrospectively proven cardiac amyloidosis causing heart failure was their increased sensitivity to digoxin.

The aetiology of these myocardial deposits of amyloid has not yet been determined. It may be degenerative, or it may be accelerated by malnutrition, or there may be other factors as yet unknown responsible for its formation. A further frustrating finding is that as yet there are no constant or typical clinical features indicating the presence of this condition.

Yet another problem in cardiac disease in the elderly is presented by endocarditis. Though a rare condition, its rarity is magnified in view of the difficulties of diagnosis. Two main types are generally recognised. Bacterial endocarditis is often missed, for the generally accepted signs and symptoms are masked or absent. Thrombotic endocarditis is seen most often in elderly patients. With this last condition the only valvular deformity may be calcification of the valve ring or cusp. The thrombi themselves are generally friable and are attached to the closure lines of the cusps. Fragments, therefore, may be easily detached and cause emboli in many sites. Thrombotic endocarditis is often associated with wasting conditions or malignancy but it has also been found in the elderly in the absence of such conditions.

The anatomy, histopathology, and electrophysiology of normal and abnormal intra-cardiac conduction, have been subjected to intense study in recent years. Rosenbaum and colleagues[10] from Buenos Aires, have established that the normal human intra-ventricular conduction system consists of three fascicles. These are: (a) the right bundle; (b) the anterior division of the left bundle; and (c) the posterior division of the same bundle. The left posterior fascicle is the most robust division, well endowed with blood vessels. The right bundle, and the anterior division of the left bundle contain the same type of fibres. They are frequently involved together in pathological processes, for the anterior division is slender and adjacent to the right bundle branch.

With the recognition of these anatomical divisions, it has been possible to determine definite electrocardiographic patterns due to involvement of the various fascicles of the left bundle. This has given rise to the concept of hemi-block which can be either anterior or posterior. Left anterior hemi-block produces left axis deviation of $-60°$ or more without significant QRS widening. Left posterior hemi-block results in strong right axis deviation of about $+120°$ and may be difficult to distinguish from right ventricular hypertrophy.

Conduction block may occur in each of these three fascicles independently, in any combination of two, or in all three simultaneously. Because of its rich blood supply, isolated block of the posterior division is rare. This is not so with the slender anterior branch, and block affecting it is now recognised as the commonest cause of left axis deviation in the electrocardiogram. In patients over 40 years of age the most frequent cause of left anterior hemi-block is anterior myocardial infarction. The presence of strong left axis deviation in patients with typical angina pectoris but without infarction is thought to be an indication of disease of the left anterior descending coronary artery.

Right bundle branch block, and left anterior hemi-block occur frequently together, due to vulnerability of these two bundles, having a shared blood supply and anatomical proximity. When both of these fascicles are involved the electrocardiogram shows left axis deviation with right bundle branch block. This most frequently occurs with anterior myocardial infarction. Two groups of elderly patients have been described as having such electrocardiographic findings and no evidence of other clinical heart disease. One group eventually proceeds to degrees of atrioventricular block, and then complete block with Stokes-Adams attacks.[4] The other group does not have such a progression.[5] The cause in the first is thought to be bilateral bundle branch fibrosis and in the second, sclerosis of the structures adjacent to the conducting system. Rosenbaum's experience demonstrates that right bundle branch block with left anterior hemi-block is common, and that 5 to 10% of people with it will eventually develop complete heart block. The much rarer combination of right bundle branch block and left posterior hemi-block, however, more consistently heralds the development of complete heart block.

Turning aside from the pathology of the elderly heart, I would like to deal now with cardiac disease as it occurs in the ambulant elderly person in the community. A randomly selected group of elderly people living at home in urban communities in the West of Scotland took part in a survey. In all they numbered 501. All responded to a standardized clinical questionnaire, had identical physical examinations and wherever possible had 13 lead electrocardiograms and standard 6 feet posteroanterior chest radiographs. Some difficulty was encountered in classifying the cardiac disorders on the basis of the information gained from the clinical history, examination and investigations. The following outline seemed most satisfactory:

(1) Definite heart disease with classifiable disorders consisting of those with clinical cardiac abnormalities or definite electrocardiographic or radiographic abnormalities.

(2) Definite but unclassifiable disorders consisting of positive cardiographic or radiological abnormalities in the absence of clinical findings.

(3) Doubtful heart disease when the subject had no clinical abnormalities and only doubtful investigative evidence of cardiac disease.

(4) No cardiac disease.

Classifiable disorders were further divided into those who have an apparent disorder of single aetiology such as ischaemic or hypertensive heart disease or those who had mixed cardiac disorders. In the series all of those falling into the mixed group had hypertensive and ischaemic heart disease combined. The terms "probable" and "possible" left ventricular hypertrophy refer to those adopted by Kannel et al.[2] with reference to electrocardiographic changes.

In these ambulant, non-hospitalised, elderly members of the community, ischaemic heart disease occurred with an incidence of 20% in men and in 12% in women (Fig. 1). A history of cardiac

DEFINITE CLASSIFIABLE HEART DISEASE

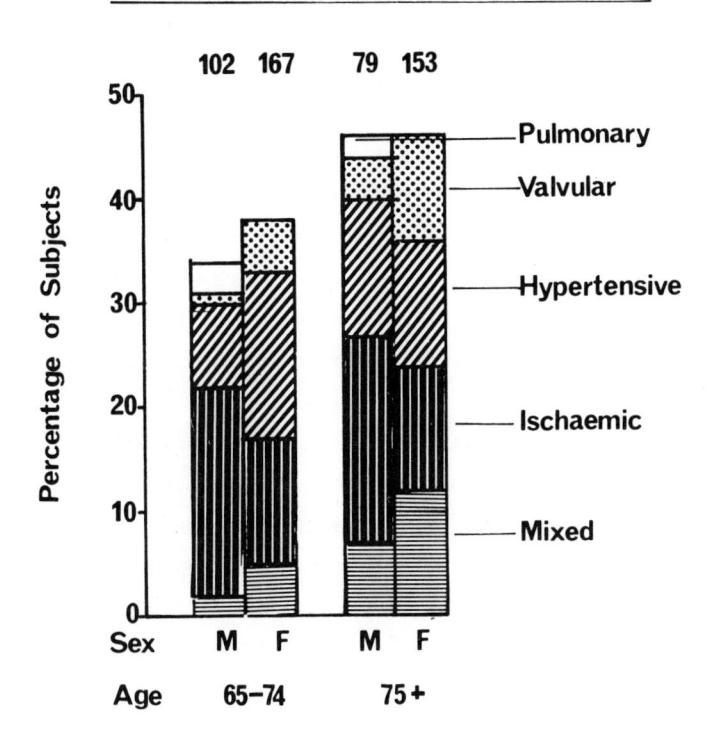

Fig. 1

pain was the most frequent index of ischaemic heart disease. However, 20% of the men and 37% of the females with ischaemic heart disease had electrocardiographic evidence of an old myocardial infarction but did not admit to having suffered previous cardiac pain. Arrhythmias occurred twice as frequently in men with ischaemic heart disease as in the similar group of women.

Hypertensive heart disease occurred next in frequency with an incidence of 16% in those women aged 65-74 and 12% in women aged 75 and over. The corresponding figures in men were 8% for the younger group and 13% for the older. Hypertensive heart disease was considered to be present when the resting blood pressure was over 180/110 mm.Hg. and the electrocardiogram showed evidence of "probable" left ventricular hypertrophy.

Valvular heart disease is known to be not uncommon in the elderly, with an incidence of approximately 4% in elderly hospital patients with mitral valve disease and about the same for aortic. The incidence in this survey of such valvular disease was slightly less than that occurring in elderly hospital patients. Both mitral valve disease and aortic valve disease were commoner in women. In this group arrhythmias occurred infrequently. Pulmonary heart disease occurred rarely and only in men. However, hypertensive and ischaemic heart disease together occurred much more frequently in the females.

Definite but unclassifiable heart disease generally meant as abnormal electrocardiogram, indicating either bundle branch block, marked evidence of arrhythmia, or probable left ventricular hypertrophy (Fig. 2). There remained a small group which was termed doubtful heart disease. This consisted of those subjects with minimally abnormal electrocardiogram or moderate increase in the cardio-thoracic ratio, without evidence of other clinical abnormality. It was difficult to decide whether people with only such slight investigative abnormalities should be regarded

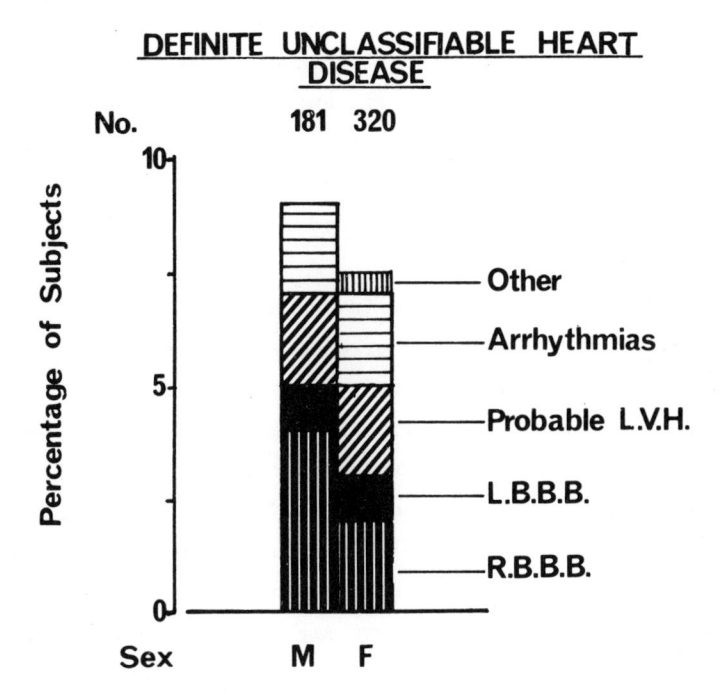

Fig. 2

as having cardiac disease. It may be, however, that some at least in this group are suffering from amyloidosis, or some other cardiomyopathy which only prolonged follow-up and postmortem examination will determine.

This survey then indicated that 40% of the elderly population in the 65-74 year old age group had evidence of definite cardiac abnormality. Only about half of those of this age had no evidence whatsoever of cardiac involvement. In the older age group, that is those of 75 years and over, only about 40% of the ambulant elderly had no evidence of cardiac upset. It was also found that in the same population less than half had normal electrocardiograms and that 23% had multiple electrocardiographic abnormalities.[3]

The anticipated increase in the elderly population will mean that more old people will require benefit from artificial pacing. Indications for a permanent pacing device in the elderly are the same as in the younger individual. The improvement achieved by the implantation of such a device in both physical and mental performance has been well documented. A small but definite number of those elderly people experiencing falls is due to either paroxysmal or permanent heart block. Treatment with long acting isoprenaline preparations may prove of benefit in some of these subjects, but most require a permanent pacing system. In some centres, patients falling within the scope of geriatric practice have undergone surgical treatment for obstructive or incompetent valvular disease. While the numbers of the elderly requiring reconstructuve valvular surgery and proving fit enough to withstand such major procedures remains small, there will with time be an ever-expanding group who will benefit from such treatment.

The ease with which toxic symptoms due to digoxin can be induced in the elderly is becoming more and more apparent, especially in those with a diminished glomerular filtration rate.

The provision of low dosage digoxin tablets has helped to reduce the number of such toxic manifestations. Serum digoxin assays, using isotopically labelled digoxin can now be used to monitor the response of those individuals susceptible, or thought to be at risk due to renal impairment, from the administration of cardiac glycosides. Though at present still largely a research laboratory technique, the application of such methods is likely to increase in view of the ease with which digoxin can induce, even at low dosage, toxic effects of a severe nature in many elderly subject.

References

1. Bedford, P.D. and Caird, F.I. (1960). Valvular disease in old age. London, J.A. Churchill.
2. Kannel, W.B., Gordon, T., Castelli, W.P. and Margolis, J.R. (1970). Electrocardiographic left ventricular hypertrophy and the risk of coronary heart disease. Ann. Int. Med., 72, 813.
3. Kennedy, R.D. and Caird, F.I. (1972). The application of the Minnesota code to population studies of the electrocardiogram in the elderly. Geront. Clin., 14, 5.
4. Lenegre, J. (1969). Etiology and pathology of bilateral bundle branch block in relation to complete heart block. Progress in Cardiovascular Disease, 6, 409.
5. Lev, M. (1964). Anatomic basis for atrioventricular block. Am. J. Med., 37, 742.
6. Pomerance, C. (1965). Senile cardiac amyloidosis. Brit. Heart J., 27, 711.
7. Pomerance, A. (1967). Ageing changes in human heart valves. Brit. Heart J., 29, 222.
8. Pomerance, A. (1972). Pathogenesis of aortic stenosis and its relation to age. Brit. Heart J., 34, 569.
9. Registrar General for Scotland (1971). Statistics, Scotland 1969. H.M.S.O.
10. Rosenbaum, M.B., Elizari, M.V. and Lazzari, J.O. (1968). Los hemibloqueos. Ed. Paidos, Buenos Aires.

ADVANCES IN NUTRITION AND SOCIOLOGY

ADVANCES IN NUTRITION AND SOCIOLOGY

Chairman's Remarks

BERNARD ISAACS

Consultant Physician
Department of Geriatric Medicine
Glasgow Royal Infirmary Group of Hospitals

A colleague seeking to establish a department of geriatric medicine was asked by the Professor of Medicine "To what discipline does the geriatrician subject himself, which entitles him to claim the status of specialist?" To this penetrating question my answer is in a word "Perception". The discipline of the geriatrician is to perceive the patient and his needs; to explore areas beyond the confines of conventional medical disciplines; to ask new questions; to seek new answers; and to arrive at new ways of giving service. This is the link between the two subjects which we have under discussion - nutrition and sociology.

The two speakers on nutrition are both noted for highly original contributions to the field. Their work and that of others was reviewed in a recent article by Berry and Darke.[1] The conventional approach to the subject of nutrition is concern with how much is eaten of what foods, and the effects on health of insufficient or excessive intake. The geriatrician perceives further elements in the nutritional situation of the elderly. The food intake of old people is an expression of perseveration or adaptation of lifelong food-behaviour patterns in the presence of the physical, psychological and social changes which inevitably occur in later life. Here are just a few of the questions to which such an approach gives rise:

To what extent does an old person's selection of foods and methods of cooking perpetuate the patterns of his childhood, and thus reflect the purchasing power, food availability and nutritional ideas of the cohort to which his parents belonged? What is the relationship between psychological change in the older person, such as fixity of mental set, and the availability of new convenience foods? Are these accepted because they are convenient or rejected because they are new? What are the effects on the quantity and type of food purchased, the method of preparation and the amount consumed of such social changes as bereavement, rise or fall of income, or eating at lunch clubs? Should nutritional improvement be sought by advice, by provision of welfare foods, by fortification, by the encouragement of communal eating? How do the problems of the next cohort of old people differ from those of the present one? Should we be urged to eat more or to eat less? Doubtless these and other matters will be touched upon by our speakers.

The field of sociology is represented by four speakers of international repute, none of whom is a sociologist. This is a bold indication of the confidence with which geriatricians move in the sociological world; they have even learned to speak the language. This is because geriatric medicine has from its birth perceived the intense interaction between physical, mental and social wellbeing. The contribution of earlier sociologists, medical and non-medical, such as the late Dr. J.H. Sheldon[3] and Professor Peter Townsend[4] to whose pioneering work we are deeply indebted, was to display the plight of those in direst need.

Today we turn our attention to the broader question of the quality of life in the later years, with special emphasis on the delivery of medical care. Permit me to draw an illustration from some recent unpublished work on dementia from my own department (Isaacs et al.)[2] In the course of a community survey we found that severe dementia afflicted some 5 or 6 per cent of the population aged 75 and over. One-half of severely demented subjects were at home, one-half in hospital. Of the factors which determined whether the subjects entered hospital or remained at home the most important was not the severity of illness but whether or not a son or daughter lived in the area. The majority of those with families close to them remained at home, while all those without children near them entered hospital.

The mentally impaired who were cared for at home fell into three equal groups, to which we gave the names "low expectation" "high toleration" and "near desperation". These reflected three distinctive patterns of reaction to the presence within the family of a mentally disturbed old person: the apathetic tolerance of those who perceived no problem; the unquestioning acceptance of a burdensome task by those to whom devotion and service were privileges; and the defeat of the spirit of those who had gone far but could go no farther in shouldering the heavy load of responsibility and care.

In future the number of demented old people in the population is unlikely to diminish. Not only will the number of the very old increase, but as yet we know of no way of arresting or preventing the pathological changes in the brain which underlie the principal types of dementia. But the structure and attitudes of society will change. Increased mobility will further diffract family structure. Improved education, housing and social services will raise expectations. Perhaps, and this is mere conjecture, but perhaps the change that many have commented on in the ethical values of society will alter our toleration of illness in the family. All these factors will work towards aggravating the pressures which illness in old age imposes on our health-care activities.

The geriatrician does wisely in equipping himself with the tools of the sociologist. In so doing he acquaints himself with the true nature of the problem confronting society, and perceives those areas where his necessarily limited resources can be most effectively deployed in the relief of human suffering.

References

1. Berry, W.T.C. and Darke, S.J. (1962). Nutrition of the elderly living at home. Age and Ageing, $\underline{i}$, 177.

2. Isaacs, B., Kennie, A.T., Arnott, M., Gunn, J.M., McQuistan, J. and Neville, Y. The ecology of dementia. To be published.

3. Sheldon, J.H. (1948). The social medicine of old age. London, Oxford University Press.

4. Townsend, P. (1957). The family life of old people. London, Routledge and Kegan Paul.

NUTRITION IN THE ELDERLY

THOMAS G. JUDGE

Consultant Physician in Geriatric Medicine
Stobhill Hospital, Glasgow

When nutritional requirements are considered in any age group, there are two standards which may be applied - the minimal and the optimal. Minimal requirements are met when an individual takes in the quantities of various nutrients which would keep an average person free from frank nutritional disease. The minimal requirements of vitamin C, for example, is 6.5 mgm. per day.[11] Obviously such an intake is likely to be inadequate in the face of increased need due for example to infection, injury or surgery. Optimal requirements are met when an individual takes in the quantities of all nutrients to maintain himself in optimum health.[3]

Sub-clinical nutritional deficiency, where the intake of one or more nutrient is inadequate for the individual concerned, is by definition lacking in specific symtoms and signs. An individual in this state, however, is readily precipitated into overt subnutrition by stress. The evidence for and against the existence of sub-clinical deficiency of various nutrients is critically reviewed in Hyam's excellent paper.[12]

Primary nutritional disease occurs when the intake of any nutrient is inadequate, for example, primary starvation occurs when calorie intake is inadequate. Secondary or conditioned sub-nutrition occurs when intake is inadequate in any individual at any time because of increased need or increased loss. Examples are the increased requirement of vitamin D in people with malabsorption, the increased need for vitamin B12 and folic acid following partial gastrectomy, the increased need for calcium magnesium when the diet is rich in phytic acid, the increased need for iron when the tetracyclines are given, because of their chalating action and the interference between the hypnotic glutethamide ("Doriden") and vitamin D.

Nutritional allowances can be calculated from population studies or from balance studies. In the case of population data, provided the sample is large and randomly selected, and that the population studied is reasonably normal, then the mean values of intake of most nutrients is likely to be normal. Balance studies are notoriously difficult but provide much more reliable information than population studies. They do however require considerable care in their application. Munro[18] derived the allowance of protein of 0.35G per kilogramme of body weight from nitrogen balance studies under ideal conditions, but he went on to suggest that older people in less artificial situations probably need 0.6G, and this appears to be the allowance that the D.H.S.S. calculations[5d] are based upon. Both population and balance studies can be misleading and it is prudent to allow a wide safety margin.

The principal sources of nutrients in the elderly are not necessarily the same as those listed in food tables which, after all, merely list nutrient content of foods: interpretation requires knowledge of eating habits. Caird and MacLeod, in their extensive and meticulously detailed study of the elderly of varying social class in Glasgow, to which I shall refer frequently,[1] show that whilst meat provides 28% of protein, as might be expected, the next common source is bread, which provides 15%, as does milk.

Calorie Requirements

There has been considerable dispute over the years about the energy requirements of older people. Table 1, based on the D.H.S.S. report of 1969[5a] is the most up-to-date authoritative reference. The D.H.S.S. survey of 1968 published in 1972[6f] found a mean calorie intake of 1,973 (8.2 MJ) with a mean energy intake in men of 2,235 kcal (9.4 MJ) compared with 1,711 kcal (7.2 MJ) in women. The main sources of energy in the diet of the elderly[1] are biscuits, cakes, pastries and bread, followed by milk, meat, fats and oils.

Protein

The dietary protein allowance recommended by the Food and Nutrition Board (USA) is 0.9G per kilogramme of body weight.[10] On this generous basis 40% of the elderly sampled in south-west Scotland had an inadequate protein intake. If the less favourable figure of 0.6G per kilo. is used, then 6 individuals in the 100 sampled in the same area failed to achieve this intake. Should this sample represent the United Kingdom as a whole, and there is no evidence to support or deny this idea, then some 360,000 old people will fail to reach this standard. On the other hand, if the standard of obtaining 10% of calories from protein is used, no one appears to be low in protein intake.

Several factors operate to lead to poor protein intake - ignorance about good protein sources such as milk, cheese and eggs for one, and the rising cost of protein for another. In 1971 a gramme of protein obtained from an egg cost 0.35p, now in late 1973 it costs 0.54p.[14]

Carbohydrate

It has frequently been assumed that obesity in the elderly is the result of spending less money on food, but as MacLeod[17]

Table 1

Age Range	Occupational Category	Body Weight kg	Energy Kcal	MJ
MEN				
65 up to 75 years	Assuming a	63	2350	9.8
75 and over	sedentary life	63	2100	8.8
WOMEN				
55 up to 75 years	Assuming a	53	2050	8.6
75 and over	sedentary life	53	1900	8.0

* 1 kilocalorie = 4.186 kilojoules.

Reproduced from Recommended Intakes of Nutrients for the United Kingdom, H.M.S.O.[5]

has shown the fat spend on average the same amount on food as do the thin; they do however buy more cheap, convenient and filling carbohydrate. This finding is confirmed in the D.H.S.S. report[6g] of a direct relationship between increasing skin-fold thickness and increasing expenditure on food. There appears to be an increased efficiency in absorbing carbohydrate with increasing age,[8] and this may be a contributory factor in the genesis of the most common disorder of nutrition in the elderly in the United Kingdom at the present time - obesity.

Fat Soluble Vitamins

Vitamin A

This substance is found preformed in milk, butter, cheese, egg yolk, liver and fatty fish, but the significant sources for the elderly are liver fats and oils. The pro-vitamin, the carotenoid pigments, are found in green, yellow and red vegetables and fruit. The serum vitamin A level ranges from 50-300 i.u., with a mean value of 148, whilst the serum carotene levels are from 15-370µG%, with a mean value of 133.[2] Serum carotene levels are raised in the elderly,[16] but although carotene/retinol block occurs in diabetes and sub-thyroidism, there is no evidence of this as yet in the elderly. Retinol (vitamin A) is stable in cooking and canning; indeed Drummond[7] in 1939 tested food packed in 1824 for the Arctic voyage of H.M.S. Heclas and found the carotene content of the carrots similar to that of fresh ones. The daily requirement of vitamin A is 2,500 i.u. (750µG of retinol) or 4,500µG of carotene or 9,000µG of other biologically active carotenoids. The D.H.S.S. report on the 1968 survey[6a] does not distinguish these three groups, but lumps retinol and the carotenoids together: the intakes found in the survey range from 3,000-4,000 i.u. It may be that this data conceals deficiency, but if so no clinical syndrome is as yet recognised.

Vitamin D

Professor Exton-Smith has dealt with this substance in his chapter; I would only add that the main sources for the elderly are eggs, fish, fats and oils, that the allowance is 2.5µG per day as cholecalciferol and that the D.H.S.S. survey reports[6b] intakes as follows:

Men: 65 - 74 3.3µG   Women: 65 - 74 2.3µG
     75+   2.7µG   75+   2.1µG

Water Soluble Vitamins

Vitamin C

Foods rich in this vitamin are fruit, brussel sprouts and potatoes[4a], but the main source for the elderly is the potato.[1] Figure 1 shows the fall-off in vitamin C level in potatoes with storage and cooking, explaining in part the seasonal variation in the incidence of scurvy.[9] The D.H.S.S. report on vitamin C intakes is reassuring[6c]; although the mean value of 39 mgm. is above the recommended level of 30 mgm., the standard deviation indicates that some individuals fail to reach this level. The Glasgow data[1] reveal the following:

Men: 65 - 74   32.3 (range 11-112.9)
       75+   31.5 (range 12.5-79.3)

Women: 65 - 74   30.1 (range 6-148)
       75+   26.5 (range 6-109).

On clinical evidence it is likely that anyone consistently taking less than 12.5 mgm. of vitamin C per day runs the risk of developing scurvy, particularly if exposed to infection or trauma.

Vitamin B complex. Riboflavine

Riboflavine is found in liver, milk, eggs and green vegetables, but in the elderly 30% of riboflavine comes from milk.[1] It is important to realise that milk exposed to sunlight - for example in a bottle on the doorstep - rapidly loses its

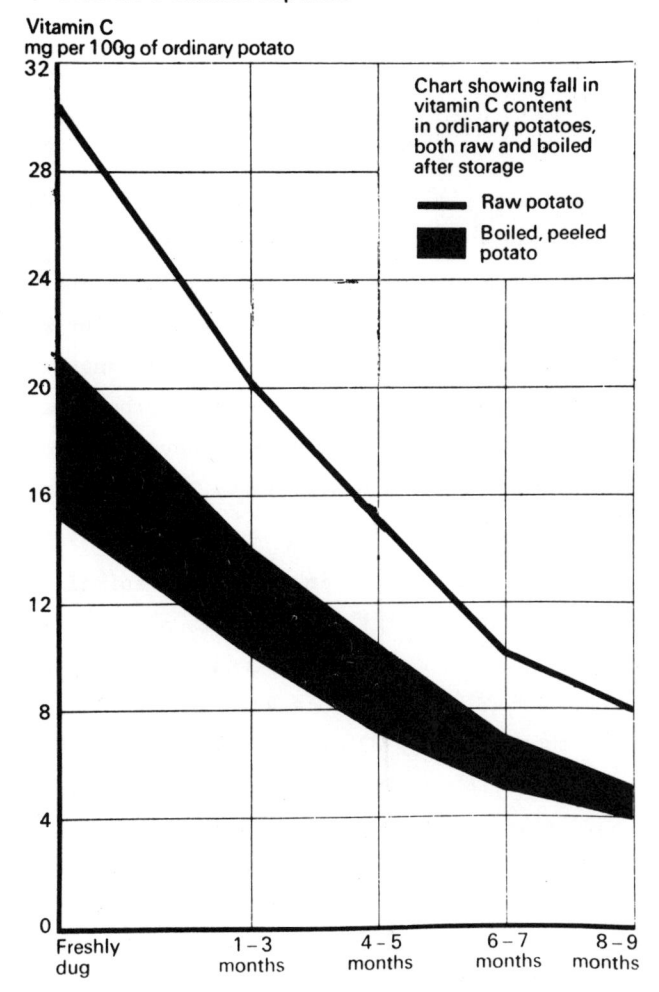

Figure 1

Reproduced by kind permission of the publishers,
The Consumers Association Ltd., from "Which",
February, 1970, p. 39.

riboflavine, and the use of cartons for milk in the elderly is strongly recommended.[6h] The allowance is 1-2 mg. per day and the Glasgow data is as follows:

   Males: 65 - 74 1.6 ± .6
        75+   1.3 ± .4
   Females: 65 - 74 1.2 ± .5
        75+   1.1 ± .4

The mean values are very similar in the D.H.S.S. 1968 study[6d] and there is considerable anxiety about the riboflavine status in many elderly patients. The average intake of milk in the United Kingdom is 10.15 oz., whereas in Glasgow the average intake is 5-9 oz. The clinical signs of riboflavine lack are angular stomatitis, chelosis, nasolabial seborrhoea and corneal vascularisation. The red tongue and the orogenital syndrome are non-specific signs of multiple vitamin deficiency.

Nicotinic Acid

Nicotinic acid is found widely in plants and animal material but the main source for the elderly is meat, from which it is lost in the dripping and glaze. It can be synthetised in the gut from Tryptophan. The allowance according to Davidson and Passmore[4c] is approximately 12 mg. a day, and from the D.H.S.S. 1969 report 15-18 mg. per day.[5b] In the D.H.S.S. 1968 study[6e] the mean intake was 13 mg. a day, and in the four age and sex groups was as follows. The Glasgow data is similar.

   Males: 65 - 74 16.8 Females: 65 - 74 11.5
      75+ 13.6   75+ 10.2

These figures are extremely worrying in the light of recommended allowances and the syndrome of nicotinic acid lack - Pellagra, the syndrome of the three D's (diarrhoea, dermatitis and dementia) or perhaps the three E's (erythema, enteritis and encephalopathy) is very important to diagnose and treat.

Thiamine

Thiamine is found in the seeds of plants and all fruit and vegetables, but the principle sources for the elderly are meat, bread and milk. The allowance is 1.4 mg. per day according to the B.M.A. recommendation[4e], and 0.8 mg. per day according to the D.H.S.S. 1969 report.[5c] In the recent D.H.S.S. report[6j] the main intake in the elderly was 0.9 mg. and the table shows the distribution by age and sex:

      Males: 65 - 74 1.1   Females: 65 - 74 .8
              75+ .9   75+ .7

These figures are worrying in terms of beri-beri which is rarely recognised. In the past we have looked for the full form of the disease characterised by high output heart failure, but there is some recent evidence suggesting that a low output varient of the disease can occur.

Vitamin B.12

As Professor Exton-Smith has pointed out, primary dietary deficiency of this vitamin is extremely rare. Indeed it is only seen in strict vegetarians and even then it is uncommon. Secondary deficiency, however, is quite common in the elderly due to the age change of atrophic gastritis resulting in increased requirements. In a recent random sample of 100 elderly subjects I found six cases of this nature. However, such a deficiency is not correctable by nutritional means.

Folic Acid

Since the precise requirements of folic acid are not known, and since food tables are unreliable, and since laboratory assessment of serum levels are unpredictable, it is difficult to be accurate on this subject. There is little doubt that in some parts of the country folate deficiency in the elderly is quite common and Table 2 shows the factors to be considered in suspected nutritional folate deficiency. From a clinical point of

Table 2

Factors to consider in suspected
nutritional folate depletion

Malabsorption

Chronic infection

Malignancy

Rheumatoid arthritis

Chronic skin disease

Chronic alcoholism

Possibly iron deficiency increasing tendency to folate depletion

Anticonvulsant drugs

Phenobarbitone (rarely)

Tuinal

Phenylbutazone

Nitrofurantoin (doubtful)

Taking of antibiotics, sulphonamides

Technical problems in Lactobacillus casei assay

Technical errors in vitamin B12 assay

Reproduced by kind permission of the author, editors and publishers of Vitamins in the Elderly. Ed. A.N. Exton-Smith and D.R. Scott "Deficiencies of Folic Acid and Vitamin B12" R.H. Girdwood, John Wright & Sons Ltd., Bristol, 1968.

view, the condition should be suspected in any unexplained neuropathy or myopathy, anaemia or confusional state.[19]

Iron

Iron deficiency anaemia is the commonest anaemia in old age, as it is in any other age. Whether or not non-anaemia sideropaenia is important is still open to doubt. There is no doubt, however, that some 40% of the elderly with normal haemoglobin have a low serum iron saturation. Poor intake of iron in those living on a tea and toast regime, coupled with increased incidence of blood loss in old age from, for example, aspirin consumption, hiatus hernia, and diverticulus disease, are the main aetiology factors in iron deficiency. Soremark[20] in Sweden has shown that the haemoglobin level in elderly subjects is directly proportional to the number of teeth whether natural or artificial, and this is a very important practical point. In the D.H.S.S. study of the elderly in the United Kingdom[6i] it was found that there was a direct relationship between the haemoglobin level and the amount of meat in the diet. Obviously it is not the total intake of iron which is important, but its availability.

Potassium

Sixty per cent of women over the age of 65 and 40% of men in their own homes have an intake of potassium of less than 60 m.eq. per day.[13] It is probable that below this level, symptoms attributable to potassium lack, develop[5], but it is certain that below 30 m.eq. per day, total body depletion rapidly follows. The principal sources of potassium in the diet are milk and citrus fruit, but these are not consumed in adequate amounts by the elderly. Symptoms of potassium lack are weakness, apathy, constipation and confusion.

Magnesium

Magnesium is widely distributed in all foods, but significant sources for the elderly are bread and milk.[1] The allowance is not known but the average British diet contains 17 to 34 m.eq. per day.[4b] The intake of elderly people in a recent random sample in Glasgow was from 19 ± 7 in women over the age of 75 to 28 ± 12 in men from 65 to 74.[1] It is probable that nutritional deficiency of magnesium does occur in some patients. The symptoms closely resemble those of potassium deficiency and the aetiological factors resemble calcium.

References

1. Caird, F.I. and MacLeod, Catriona. Department of Geriatric Medicine, University of Glasgow. Personal communication.
2. Campbell, D.A. and Tonks, E.L. (1962). Biochemical findings in human retinitis pigmentosa with particular reference to vitamin A deficiency. Brit. J. Ophthal., 46, 151.
3. Darke, Sylvia (1972). Requirements for vitamins in old age. In: Nutrition in Old Age. Ed. Lars A. Carlson. Almqvist and Wiksell, Stockholm, p. 107.
4. Davidson, Sir S. and Passmore, R. (1966). Human Nutrition and Dietetics. 3rd Ed., Livingstone, Edinburgh.
    - a) Vitamin C, p. 209.
    - b) Magnesium, p. 159.
    - c) Nicotinic Acid, p. 216.
    - d) Thiamine, p. 215.
    - e) Thiamine, p. 240.
5. Department of Health and Social Security (1969). Recommended Intakes of Nutrients for the United Kingdom. H.M.S.O., London.
    - a) Calories, p. 4.
    - b) Nicotinic Acid, p. 4.
    - c) Thiamine, p. 4.
    - d) Protein, p. 16.
6. Department of Health and Social Security (1972). A Nutrition Survey of the Elderly. H.M.S.O., London.
    - a) Vitamin A, p. 17.
    - b) Vitamin D, p. 17.
    - c) Vitamin C, p. 17.
    - d) Riboflavine, p. 17.
    - e) Nicotinic Acid, p. 17.
    - f) Calories, p. 25.
    - g) Skinfold thickness, p. 27.
    - h) Cartons, p. 55.
    - i) Iron, p. 58.
    - j) Thiamine, p. 17.

7   Drummond, J.C. and Lewis, W.R. (1939). Examination of some tinned food of historic interest. Chem & Ind., 57, 808.

8   Durnin, J.V. (1966). Age, physical activity and energy expenditure. Proc. Nutr. Soc., 25, 107.

9   Dymock, I. Department of Medicine, University of Manchester. Personal communication.

10 Food and Nutrition Board (1968). Recommended Dietary Allowances. 7th Ed. National Academy of Sciences. National Research Council Publication, 1964, Washington.

11 Hodges, R.E., Baker, E.M., Hood, J., Sauberlich, H.E. and March, S.C. (1969). Experimental scurvy in man. Amer. J. Clin. Nutr., 22, 535.

12 Hyams, D.E. (1973). Nutrition of the Elderly. Mod. Geriatrics, 3, 7, 356.

13 Judge, T.G. (1968). Hypokalaemia in the elderly. Geront. Clin., 10, 102.

14 Judge, T.G. (1971). Eat Well and Keep Well. Med. News Tribune.

15 Judge, T.G. (1972). Potassium metabolism in the elderly. In: Nutrition in Old Age. Ed. Lars A. Carlson, Almqvist and Wiksell, Stockholm, p. 86.

16 McLennan, W.J. (1971). Xylose absorption and serum carotene levels in the elderly. Geront. Clin., 13, 370.

17 MacLeod, Catriona (1970). Dietary intake of older people. Nutrition, 24, 24.

18 Munro, H.N. (1972). Protein requirements and metabolism in ageing. In: Nutrition in Old Age. Ed. Lars A. Carlson. Almqvist and Wiksell, Stockholm, p. 32.

19 Sneath, P., Chanarin, I., Hodkinson, H.M., McPherson, C.K. and Reynolds, E.H. (1973). Folate studies in a geriatric population and its relation to dementia. Age and Ageing, 2, 3, 177.

20 Soremark, R. and Nilsson, B. (1972). Dental status and nutrition in old age. In: Nutrition in Old Age. Ed. Lars A. Carlson. Almqvist and Wiksell, Stockholm, p. 147.

VITAMINS AND THE ELDERLY

A.N. EXTON-SMITH

Professor of Geriatric Medicine
University College Hospital

A diagnosis of malnutrition was made in 3% of the elderly population surveyed in the study sponsored by the Department of Health and Social Security.[13] The clinical diagnosis included both protein-calorie malnutrition and specific vitamin deficiencies. Rarely, however, was there a primary cause associated with environmental or economic factors. In the majority of cases an underlying medical condition was discovered to account for the malnutrition. Thus the problem of malnutrition in this age group is largely related to that of ascertainment of the other unmet medical and social needs of old people. In recent years considerable attention has been paid to the investigation of the prevalence of vitamin deficiencies in the elderly population; surveys have been conducted in groups of old people living at home, in residents of old people's homes and in geriatric wards of hospitals.

Detection of Malnutrition

An important aim of nutritional surveys is to gain information on the nutritional status of the individuals concerned.

If the subjects included in the survey are a random sample of the elderly population it is possible to assess the extent of nutritional deficiencies in the older sections of the community. Malnutrition may be defined as a disturbance of form or function due to lack of (or excess of) calories or of one or more nutrients.[21] A diagnosis cannot be made on the sole finding of a low dietary intake; but when there are specific clinical signs of malnutrition associated with low intake of nutrients then a dietary origin of malnutrition must be strongly suspected.

In a survey sponsored by the King Edward's Fund in 1965[19] an investigation was made of the diets of old people living alone at home in two North London boroughs. The group selected was 60 women whose ages ranged from 70-80 years (with the exception of 3 aged 89, 90 and 94 years). The mean daily intakes of nutrients were satisfactory and are shown in Table 1.

Only a few instances of nutritional deficiency were revealed by the survey. There was, however, a striking correlation between diet and health; nearly all the subjects whose diet was better than average were judged on clinical assessment to be better than average in health. This does not necessarily mean that good diet is responsible for good health, since the reverse might equally be true in that better health and physical activity might be associated with good appetite and a larger intake of food.

When the 60 subjects were arranged in groups according to their ages there was found to be a striking decrease in intakes of all nutrients with advancing age. The percentage falls in intake for subjects in their late seventies compared with those in their early seventies are shown in Table 2.

In spite of the considerable reduction in nutrient intake with age there seemed to be little alteration in the quality of the diet. Thus the percentage of calories derived from protein

Table 1

Mean daily intakes of nutrients
of women in the eighth decade

Calories	1890 kcal.	Calcium	860 mg.
Protein	57 g.	Iron	9.9 mg.
Fat	74 g.	Vitamin C	37 mg.
Carbohydrate	221 g.	Vitamin D	135 i.

Table 2

Cross-sectional study: fall in intake
of nutrients during the eighth decade

Calories and Nutrients	Fall in Intake %
Calories	19
Protein	24
Fat	30
Carbohydrate	8
Calcium	18
Iron	29
Vitamin C	31

was 12.2% for the subjects in their early seventies and 11.4% for those in their late seventies.

This study reveals differences between the age groups which might be the result of several factors:

(1) True age changes affecting all individuals and leading to a reduction in physiological requirements. It is known that lean body mass and basal metabolic rate decrease with age.[2]

(2) Reduction in appetite or energy expenditure in some of the subjects due to the development of disease or physical disabilities as they enter the second half of the eighth decade. Sheldon[32] has drawn attention to the striking increase in prevalence of incapacity in the elderly population after the age of 75.

(3) Secular differences between the two groups in that the lifelong dietary pattern of the older group may have been different from that of the early seventies group. Indeed it is possible that the dietary pattern may have been a factor responsible for the longevity of those who reach extreme old age.

(4) The failure of certain individuals, notably the obese, to reach extreme old age. The late seventies group being thinner would be expected to have a lower dietary intake.

From this study it was impossible to ascertain the relative importance of these factors and it was therefore decided to conduct a follow-up study of the 60 elderly women to form a longitudinal investigation. 22 of the 60 women who participated in the first King Edward's Hospital Fund Survey were followed up $6\frac{1}{2}$ years later.[35] It was found that for those subjects who maintained their health (as assessed on clinical examination and by a scoring system recording physical disabilities) the intakes of nutrients in the two surveys were remarkably similar.

But for those women whose health had declined there was a considerable fall in intake amounting to 20% for protein and 17% for calories.

From this limited study it was concluded that nutrient intakes in old age are usually maintained provided the person remains active and fit. It was also evident that physical disabilities are often responsible for declining intakes in old age. It is therefore necessary when carrying out dietary surveys in this age group to include a medical examination of the subjects to distinguish between primary and secondary causes of malnutrition.[17]

Specific Vitamin Deficiencies

Specific tests including biochemical, haematological and radiological investigations often reveal small departures from normality and these can be related to low intakes of certain vitamins. There is evidence of low blood levels or tissue stores of vitamins in some sections of the elderly population. Thus Kataria and his colleagues[26] showed that the vitamin C status as measured by the leucocyte ascorbic acid levels was lower in old people living in residential homes and in elderly patients in hospital compared with those old people living at home in the community. Griffiths and others[23] showed that compared with a large number of younger volunteers 58% of geriatric patients on admission to hospital had low plasma ascorbic acid levels, 40% were deficient in thiamine, as measured by the transketolase test, and 24% were deficient in both. They also showed that low blood levels could be raised to those of the younger volunteers by 3 weeks vitamin supplementation. The inferior nutritional status of old people in residential homes and of patients admitted to geriatric wards can almost certainly be related to their frailty and ill-health and this situation has not necessarily any bearing on that found in fitter old people living in their own

Vitamin B Complex

A high incidence of changes in the mucous membranes of the tongue and lips associated with B complex deficiency have been described.[9,23] The classical sign of nicotinic acid deficiency is a raw 'beef-red' tongue and riboflavin deficiency leads to angular stomatitis, magenta tongue and seborrhoea of the naso-labial folds. But some of these changes can also occur in iron deficiency and vitamin B12 deficiency, following the administration of broad spectrum antibiotics and as a result of oral infection with candida albicans. The commonest cause of angular stomatitis in the elderly is the ill-fitting of dentures.

There is conflict of opinion on the extent to which abnormal tongue signs can be corrected by vitamin supplementation. Dymock and Brocklehurst[14] repeated their earlier studies and used single vitamin supplementation instead of a multi-vitamin preparation on 77 old people in hospital who survived for the one year's clinical trial. Riboflavin therapy was associated with significant improvement, and nicotinamide produced an improvement in the dorsum of the tongue. MacLeod[27] on the other hand, failed to confirm these findings. In a series of 80 patients with abnormal tongue appearance vitamin supplementation for one year had no effect on the tongue changes or the signs of angular stomatitis. Similar negative results were obtained in the series investigated by Berry and Darke.[8] Thus of the 27 patients who had lesions of the lip or angle of the mouth, 24 did not improve after one year's administration of a riboflavin containing preparation.

Moreover, in the 66 elderly patients who had abnormal appearances of the dorsum of the tongue there was no statistical difference in the response rate between those who received vitamin B supplementation and those who were treated with a placebo tablet. In 90% of the subjects who had changes in the dorsal surface of the tongue a fungal infection was found and Berry and Darke consider that this is the most likely cause of these changes.

In the nutrition study sponsored by the Department of Health and Social Security[13] carried out in 6 centres in the British Isles and employing a random sample of the elderly population in the areas, a special attempt was made to relate changes in mucous membranes to riboflavin deficiency. Of the 778 subjects examined 57 were diagnosed as having either angular stomatitis or cheilosis. The riboflavin intake of those with these lip lesions was 1.2 mgms. per day compared with a mean intake of 1.3 mgms. per day for those without these lip lesions; these differences are not statistically significant. Out of the 23 subjects who had very low intakes of riboflavin (less than 0.7 mgms. for males and 0.55 mgms. for females) 4 subjects had lip lesions. Thus, although there may be some element of clinical ariboflavinosis in the elderly population, these numbers must be very small and in general the riboflavin status appeared to be satisfactory. It is apparent that there is a discrepancy between the clinical findings and the expectation based on low dietary intakes of riboflavin.

In the study of accidental hypothermia in the elderly conducted in a random sample of the elderly population of Camden during the winter months of 1972 a limited investigation of the nutritional status of the subjects was made. In 128 subjects who attended hospital for clinical examination and other tests Thurnhaus[37] measured the erythrocyte glutathione reductase activity (EGR) and the percentage stimulation of EGR by flavin adenine dinucleotide (FAD). A stimulation of greater than 30% was found in 18% of the males and in 19% of the females. Thus it is considered that there may be marginal riboflavin deficiency in about one-fifth of the elderly population. However, the true clinical significance of low riboflavin levels (and of other vitamins) is at present not known.

A similar uncertainty exists about the exact levels of folic acid in the serum or red cells which are considered to be adequate. Herbert[24] maintains that folic acid deficiency is the commonest vitamin deficiency in men. Although a folate-free diet quickly leads to lowering of the serum folate levels, many months elapse before clinical or haematological changes develop. In a survey of elderly patients admitted to the geriatric department of the South Western Hospital, London, Hurdle and Picton Williams[25] found serum folate levels of less than 5 ng/ml in 39% of consecutive admissions. Read and his colleagues[31] in Bristol found that 80% of 50 entrants to old people's homes had folate deficiency, which they took as a level of less than 6 ng/ml. Such lower limits, however, do not represent very strict criteria of deficiency. Batata et al.[7] in Oxford adopted a lower limit of normal of 2.1 ng/ml. and found that 10% of patients over the age of sixty admitted to hospital had levels below this limit. A nutritional origin was suspected since with severe physical disability (and in consequence inability of the patient to look after himself) the more likely was there to be folate deficiency; there was found to be a statistically significant correlation between organic brain disease and low folate levels. Girdwood[22] adopting similar criteria (serum levels of less than 2.2 ng/ml.) found that 8% of elderly hospital patients in Edinburgh were deficient although he was unable to trace any cases of megaloblastic anaemia in the elderly due to nutritional deficiency. He therefore concludes that there must be considerable variation in different parts of the country; in some parts at least, megaloblastic anaemia certainly exists and there must be a reservoir of old people in Great Britain who suffer from a folate deficiency state without being significantly anaemic.[22] Although anaemia may be uncommon these deficiency states may have other adverse effects on health. Strachan and Henderson[36] have described cases of severe dementia due to folate deficiency; treatment with folic acid led to a complete resolution of the dementing process. The majority of cases of dementia are so unresponsive to treatment that the finding of a few cases of reversible dementia merits a much closer investigation into the relationship between mental impairment and folic acid metabolism.

Vitamin C

Although scurvy is now a rare disease, occasional cases are found amongst the elderly, especially in men. The manifestations include weakness, anaemia, swelling and bleeding of the gums, 'sheet' haemorrhages in the skin of the arms and legs, and sometimes haemorrhages at other sites. Sublingual 'petachiae' have been regarded as an early sign of vitamin C deficiency, but Andrews and his colleagues[4] have shown by histological examination that these lesions are usually not haemorrhages but small aneurysmal dilatations of the minute vessels under the tongue. They do not disappear when the vitamin C intake is increased and it is unlikely therefore that they are due to acute vitamin C deficiency.

It seems likely that the bodily stores of vitamin C in many old people are diminished and low levels of leucocyte ascorbic acid have been reported by several observers; the levels are lower in the elderly than in younger subjects,[10] lower in winter than in summer,[5] and lower in men than in women.[1] In a recent study Milne and his colleagues[29] measured the leucocyte ascorbic acid (LAA) levels and the vitamin C intakes in a random sample of 204 men and 247 women ($23.88 \mu g/10^8$ cells) were found to be significantly higher than for men ($18.11 \mu g/10^8$ cells). The values decreased with increasing age in women but not in men. They were significantly higher in both sexes in the six months July to December. 50% of men and 58% of women had intakes of less than 30 mg. daily, 23.6% of men and 28.1% of women have intakes of less than 20 mg. daily and 4.7% of men and 3% of women intakes less than 10 mg. daily. A significantly greater proportion of both men and women had mean intakes of less than 30 mg. daily in the months October to March compared with the months April to September. A moderate correlation was present between vitamin C intake and L.A.A. level. It was also found that L.A.A. levels increase in parallel with but lag behind seasonal increases in vitamin C intakes.

The Edinburgh study and other dietary surveys disclose that there is an appreciable number of old people who have an intake of less than 10 mg. daily which is known to be the amount required to prevent or cure scurvy.[6] A high proportion of the elderly population are consuming less than the allowance of 30 mg. per day recommended by the Department of Health and Social Security in 1969;[12] this allowance takes into account the changes in requirements due to stress and the considerable individual variations in requirements which are known to exist.[34] The majority of people will not suffer from any ill-effects from a vitamin C intake of less than 30 mg., but our assessment is handicapped through a lack of information of the levels of L.A.A. required for the maintenance of health. Windsor and Williams[39] have attempted to determine the significance of low L.A.A. levels by measuring the total hydroxyproline excretion (THP) in the urine of elderly subjects with differing vitamin C status. THP is a measure of collagen metabolism and vitamin C is required for collagen synthesis. It was found that in old people with L.A.A. levels of less than $15 \mu g/10^8$ wbc the administration of vitamin C produced a rise in THP excretion, whereas this did not occur when the L.A.A. content was greater than $15 \mu g/10^8$ wbc. It is reasonable to suppose that subclinical or clinical deficiency exists in people with L.A.A. levels of less than $15 \mu g/10^8$ wbc and there is evidence from studies in which this parameter has been measured that levels below this lower limit are commonly found in old people.

Thus Thurnham[37] in an investigation of the old people who participated in the Camden Survey of accidental hypothermia found that 28% of the men and 10% of the women had L.A.A. levels equal to or less than 15 mg/10^8 wbc. The much higher proportion of men with low levels is in keeping with the findings of the Edinburgh and other surveys and accords with clinical experience that men are more prone to scurvy than women.

Wilson and his colleagues[38] in Cornwall have reported the relationship between L.A.A. levels and mortality in the aged. Determination of L.A.A. was made on 159 patients admitted to a geriatric department. It was found that the mortality within the first 4 weeks in hospital was 47% for those whose L.A.A. level on admission was less than 12 mg/10^8 wbc, compared with 10% when the initial L.A.A. was greater than 25 µg/10^8 wbc ($p<0.01$). This significant difference in mortality between the high and low L.A.A. groups might be related to severity of illness or special clinical features. Wilson and his colleagues found no marked difference in clinical features (the incidence of such conditions as cerebrovascular disease, congestive heart failure and malignant disease being similar in the two groups), but the overall severity of the illness appeared to be greater in the group with low L.A.A. levels. Thus from this study it was not possible to say whether the vitamin C status influenced mortality directly or whether the severity of illness affected both the nutritional status and mortality. As it is believed that low L.A.A. levels can be raised by the administration of vitamin C, it will be interesting to determine whether vitamin C supplementation which Wilson proposes will affect subsequent mortality.

Vitamin D

At present the majority of cases of vitamin D deficiency are only recognised at an advanced stage when the typical biochemical findings or bone changes of osteomalacia have developed.

Recently Nordin[30] has suggested that vitamin D lack may further impair calcium absorption which is often already reduced in old age and this in turn may be responsible for osteoporosis. Thus mild long continued vitamin D deficiency may account for the increased porosity of bone in old age and the liability to fracture especially in elderly women.

Deficiency of vitamin D may be the result of several causes and those which are most commonly found in old age are:
(i) dietary lack;
(ii) inadequate exposure to sunlight;
(iii) malabsorption syndromes (including postgastrectomy states, gluten enteropathy and possibly small bowel ischaemia);
(iv) liver and biliary tract diseases;
(v) renal disease.

Several of these factors sometimes operate together; for example, mild degrees of malabsorption occurring in an old person who is housebound and having a low dietary intake.

The occurrence of vitamin D deficiency due to low dietary intake was assessed in the first King Edward's Hospital Fund survey.[19] Following the dietary investigations three-quarters of the elderly women agreed to participate in further studies involving clinical assessment, biochemical investigations and the determination of the radiographic density of bone.[18] Slightly more than one-quarter of the subjects were found to have marked skeletal rarefaction and when these subjects were compared with age-matched individuals whose bones were of higher density it was found that the former had significantly lower vitamin D intakes. Moreover, vitamin D intakes were correlated with alterations in the serum levels of calcium, inorganic phosphorus and alkaline phosphatase. Thus the findings of this study suggest that dietary vitamin D deficiency may contribute to the skeletal rarefaction which is so common in old age.

Smith and his colleagues[33] in the United States assessed the vitamin D status of a group of women living in Michigan (average age 60.6 years) and compared them with a group of women of similar age living in Puerto Rico. For the Michigan group the level of vitamin D in the blood (serum anti-rachitic activity) was significantly lower in those subjects with low bone density compared with those having normal bones and the level showed marked seasonal variation. By contrast, in Puerto Rico, where there is much greater exposure to sunlight and a higher vitamin D content of the food, the incidence of skeletal rarefaction was much lower, the serum vitamin D levels were much higher and there was no seasonal variation. The authors attributed the skeletal rarefaction to osteoporosis, rather than to osteomalacia, but they noted a correlation between the vitamin D levels and the serum calcium, inorganic phosphorus and alkaline phosphatase.

Clinical osteomalacia may not be rare in certain sections of the elderly population. Thus Anderson and his colleagues[3] in Glasgow found 16 cases after thorough investigation of 100 women admitted to a geriatric department and who had a possible clinical indication, namely, vague and generalised pain, bone tenderness, low backache, muscle weakness and stiffness, waddling gait, skeletal deformity, malabsorption states, long confinement indoors or malnutrition. Subsequently 100 admissions to the female geriatric wards were investigated and the incidence of osteomalacia was found to be 4% of all elderly women. The authors considered the osteomalacia to be due mainly to dietary lack of vitamin D and to unsufficient synthesis in the skin due to inadequate exposure to sunlight.

The importance of vitamin D deficiency in the causation of fractures and other orthopaedic problems in the elderly has been recognised by Chalmers and his colleagues.[11] They have described the clinical features of 37 patients with osteomalacia and the majority were elderly women. They emphasise the need for thorough screening of all elderly patients presenting with weakness, skeletal pain, pathological fractures, or with diminished radiographic density of bone. They attributed the osteomalacia to dietary deficiency of vitamin D, inadequate exposure to sunlight and mild degrees of malabsorption occurring alone or in combination.

The difficulties inherent in the detection of vitamin D deficiency in old age are immense and these problems have been discussed elsewhere.[15] It is clearly desirable to look more diligently for cases of osteomalacia amongst the elderly population and undoubtedly many cases of dietary origin will be discovered. The importance lies in the fact that the condition is so readily preventable by increased vitamin D intake and the disease when it is recognised responds most satisfactorily to simple treatment. Particular attention must be paid to the housebound who probably represent the largest single vulnerable group. The recent study of housebound old people[20] has disclosed that 48% of housebound women aged 70 to 79 years have a vitamin D intake of less than 30 i.u. per day compared with 13% of active women of similar age. For those confined to the house lack of exposure to sunlight is a significant additional factor. Moreover, if Nordin's hypothesis[30] is correct concerning the relationship betwee vitamin D deficiency and osteoporosis the problem is even greater in magnitude and more complex than has hitherto been supposed. The true extent of the problem will only be known when the importance of nutritional factors in the epidemiology of fractures in old age has been fully investigated.

Prevention of Vitamin Deficiency

The factors leading to nutritional deficiencies in old age have been discussed elsewhere. Primary dietary insufficiency can arise from ignorance, social isolation, loneliness, depression, mental impairment, physical disabilities, poverty and badly planned dietary regimes which may be continued by the patient for years longer than necessary. Secondary causes of malnutrition are even more important in the elderly than in other age groups and they include impairment of appetite, poor dentition, malabsorption, malignant and other wasting diseases, interference with the metabolism of vitamins by drugs and in some instances an increased requirement for certain nutrients. Several factors, both primary and secondary, often operate together to produce malnutrition in the individual and sometimes these factors are inter-related. Thus limited mobility, loneliness, social isolation and depression are all found in housebound old people and make them especially vulnerable when they are receiving insufficient support from relatives, friends or the community services.

Vulnerable Groups

Old people especially at risk are the recently bereaved, the socially isolated (especially those with impairment of the special senses), those with mental disorders, very old people, and those who have not consulted their general practitioners for 6 months or more. Unless these vulnerable groups of old people can be recognised, preventive measures would have to be applied to all old people irrespective of the fact that the majority will never suffer from nutritional deficiencies. The inefficiency and the undesirability of employing such procedures can only be overcome by identification of those especially at risk. The application of preventive measures to these smaller groups rather than to the whole elderly population becomes a manageable proposition.

We now believe that the housebound form the largest single group at risk. As a result of a recent investigation of the dietary and state of health of housebound old people[20] it has been shown that their vitamin C and vitamin D intakes (as well as the intakes of other nutrients) are substantially lower than those of active old people of comparable age. Physical and mental disability in old age not only affect the mode of living of those afflicted but also lead to alterations in their dietary pattern and nutritional status. The prevention of malnutrition in this group should present less difficulty than for other vulnerable groups of old people who cannot be so readily indentified since the majority of the housebound are known to the health and social services.

Improving Nutrition

Having identified the groups of old people especially at risk the individual's nutritional status must be assessed and if a dietary insufficiency is found, means must be sought for improving his nutrient intake. The assessment of dietary intakes should ideally be made by dietitians, but their skills are rarely available for old people at home. Simple scoring systems have been devised[28] and these are usually based on the number of main meals and the frequency of consumption of certain foods containing protein (meat, cheese, eggs, bread and milk). Such a system can be readily applied by a health visitor to give a rough guide on the quality of the diet.

Possible means of improving the nutrient intake of old people at home have been discussed elsewhere.[16] In brief, they included encouraging those old people who are able to do so to eat at a club in the company of others and for less active (especially the housebound) to provide an efficient meals-on-wheels service at least 5 days per week. Ignorance about food and of what constitutes a balanced diet is very common amongst the elderly, especially widowers, and to remedy this instruction must be given by dietitians or health visitors.

The most satisfactory means of improving nutrition is by improving the quality, and in some instances, the quantity of the diet. The very low intakes of certain vitamins, notably vitamins C and D must lead to consideration of the possibility of supplementation. Thus for those whose consumption of vitamin C is inadequate, intake should be improved by the addition to the diet of citrus fruit, blackcurrant juice, rose hip syrup or tomatoes.

The alternative method of increasing intake by the prescription of vitamin C tablets is satisfactory but less desirable. Similar considerations apply to riboflavin and to folic acid but the extent to which the subjects would benefit from raising the serum or tissue levels of these vitamins is doubtful.

In the case of vitamin D there is known to be considerable individual variation in requirements and since in some persons moderately excessive intakes can lead to vitamin D intoxication widespread supplementation could be harmful. A means of increasing the intake would be by the fortification of milk which is a procedure adopted in the United States, but the distribution of fortified milk would best be restricted to housebound old people for whom the intake of vitamin D is often low and the synthesis of vitamin D in the skin is inadequate through lack of exposure to sunlight.

The policy of introducing supplementation should only be decided after the results of carefully controlled experiments are available to assess the benefits of increased intakes. Once the practice of supplementation has become widespread, it is difficult to prove or assess the benefits. Moreover, there is an understandable reluctance to withdraw a prophylactic measure on the basis of doubts about its value when it has been practised for several years.

References

1. Allen, M.A., Andrews, J. and Brook, M. (1967). Nutr. Diet, 21, 136.
2. Allen, T.H., Anderson, E.C. and Langham, W.H. (1966). J. Geront., 15, 348.
3. Anderson, I., Campbell, A.E.R., Dunn, A. and Runciman, J.B.M. (1966). Scot. med. J., 11, 429.
4. Andrews, J., Letcher, M. and Brook, M. (1969). Brit. med. J., ii, 416.
5. Andrews, J., Brook, M. and Allen, M.A. (1966). Brit. med. J., 8, 257.
6. Bartley, W., Krebs, H.A. and O'Brien, J.R.P. (1953). Vitamin C requirements of human adults, Special Report Series. Medical Research Council. No. 280. H.M.S.O., London.
7. Batata, M., Spray, G.H., Bolton, F.G., Higgins, G. and Wollner, L. (1967). Brit. med. J., 2, 667.
8. Berry, W.T.C. and Darke, S.J. (1972). Age and Ageing, 1, 177.
9. Brocklehurst, J., Griffiths, L.L., Taylor, G.F., Marks, J. and Scott, D.L. (1968). Geront. Clin. (Basel) 10, 309.
10. Brook, M. and Grimshaw, J.J. (1968). Amer. J. Clin. Nutr., 21, 1254.
11. Chalmers, J., Conacher, W.D.H., Gardner, D.L. and Scott, P.J. (1967). J. Bone Jt surgery., 49B, 403.
12. Department of Health and Social Security (1969). Recommended intakes of nutrients for the United Kingdom. Reports on Public Health and Medical Subjects, No. 120, H.M.S.O., London.
13. Department of Health and Social Security (1972). Nutrition of the elderly., H.M.S.O., London.
14. Dymock, S. and Brocklehurst, J. (1972). Paper given at meeting of British Geriatrics Society, London.
15. Exton-Smith, A.N. (1968). In: Vitamins in the Elderly (Ed. by Exton-Smith, A.N. and Scott, D.L.) Wright, Bristol.

16 Exton-Smith, A.N. (1968). Roy. Soc. Health J., **88**, 205.
17 Exton-Smith, A.N. (1970). Nutrition, Lond., **24**, 218.
18 Exton-Smith, A.N., Hodkinson, H.M. and Stanton, B.R. (1966). Lancet, **ii**, 999.
19 Exton-Smith, A.N. and Stanton, B.R. (1965). An investigation of the dietary of elderly women living alone. King Edward's Hospital Fund, London.
20 Exton-Smith, A.N., Stanton, B.R. and Windsor, A.C.M. (1972). Nutrition of housebound old people. King Edward's Hospital Fund, London.
21 First Report of the Panel on the Nutrition of the Elderly (1970). Reports on Public Health and Medical Subjects, No. 123, H.M.S.O., London.
22 Girdwood, R.H. (1968). In: Vitamins in the Elderly (Ed. by Exton-Smith, A.N. and Scott, D.L.) John Wright and Sons, Bristol.
23 Griffiths, L.L., Brocklehurst, J.C., Scott, D.L., Marks, J. and Blackley, J. (1967). Geront. clin., **9**, 1.
24 Herbert, V. (1967). Am. J. clin. Nutr., **20**, 562.
25 Hurdle, A.D.F. and Williams, T.C.P. (1966). Brit. med. J., **2**, 202.
26 Kataria, M.S., Rao, D.B. and Curtis, R.C. (1965). Geront. clin., **7**, 189.
27 MacLeod, R.D. (1972). Age and Ageing, **1**, 99.
28 Marr, J., Heady, J.A. and Morris, J. (1961). Proc. 3rd Int. Congress Dietetics, London.
29 Milne, J.S., Lonergan, M.E., Williamson, J., Moore, F.M.L., McMaster, R. and Percy, N. (1971). Brit. med. j., **iv**, 383.
30 Nordin, B.E.C. (1971). Brit. med. J., **i**, 571.
31 Read, A.E., Gough, K.R., Pardoe, J.L. and Nicholas, A. (1965). Brit. med. J., **ii**, 843.
32 Sheldon, J.H. (1948). The Social Medicine of Old Age. Oxford University Press, London.
33 Smith, R.W., Rizek, J., Frame, B. and Mansour, J. (1964). Amer. J. Clin. Nutr., **14**, 98.
34 Srikantia, S.G., Mohanram, M. and Krishnaswamy, K. (1970). Amer. J. clin. Nutr., **23**, 59.
35 Stanton, B.R. and Exton-Smith, A.N. (1970). A longitudinal study of the dietary of elderly women. King Edward's Hospital Fund, London.

36 Strachan, R.W. and Henderson, J.G. (1967). Quart. J. Med., 36, 189.

37 Thurnhaus, D. (1972). Personal Communication.

38 Wilson, T.S., Weeks, M.M., Mukherjee, S.K., Murrell, J.S. and Andrews, C.T. (1972). Geront. clin. (Basel) 14, 17.

39 Windsor, A.C.M. and Williams, C.B. (1970). Brit. med. J., i, 731.

PREVENTIVE ASPECTS OF GERIATRICS

NAIRN R. COWAN

Consultant Physician
Department of Geriatric Medicine
Stobhill Hospital*

In this short account of the preventive aspects of geriatrics I propose, since casework is highly topical and relevent, to dwell mainly on the psycho-social difficulties of the aged.

Emotional disturbance, chronic physical illness, economic deprivation, society's concept of old people, reality, the meaning of work and retirement, the inability to define health with precision, the inadequacy of chronologic age as a measure of ageing, and the relative immaturity of our medico-social services are some of the more important aspects of the ageing process and there are four significant practical problems. The first is that in medical and other practices which involve human relationships lack of knowledge of the mechanics of human behaviour or sheer lack of ability can make it impossible for professional workers to evaluate successfully psycho-social illness. When a worker is unable to understand personal needs as well as the needs of the patient or client there can be lack of acceptance and desire to

---

* Lately Medical Officer of Health, Rutherglen

care for ill old people. The second problem is the disparity between the volume of old people's needs and the inadequate numbers of workers available to cope with these needs. The third facet is the "iceberg" phenomenon, that is, much disease - physical, mental and social - in the elderly is unknown to the community and remains untreated. This is aggravated by the tendency for old people to seek professional advice late rather than early in the evolution of illness, and the reasons are varied. Disease may be without symptoms or erroneously regarded as part of the normal ageing process. The fear of knowing what is going on in the body may make an individual delay assessment for as long as possible, while relatives fearful of the outcome may dissuade the aged from seeking professional guidance. Furthermore, socially isolated old people who live alone may have real difficulty in obtaining aid, while the reality of the situation may be denied, and when this denial has to be discarded by the increasing intensity of illness a serious crisis situation is likely to occur. Fourthly there is need for improved integration of effort by professional and voluntary workers.

The Rutherglen Consultative Health Centre for older people has been described elsewhere.[1] In Rutherglen surveys it has been found that the prevalence of mental illness is disturbingly high and this finding has been validated by work at Kilsyth. In a series of 1,500 people, aged 60 to 89 years, 438 men and 429 women were regarded as physically healthy while 328 men and 305 women were found to have physical disease. The incidence of serious emotional disturbance in these 4 groups was 13.5%, 18.9%, $32\frac{1}{2}$9% and 39.0% respectively and depression was the common finding. The main causes of the observed mental illness were physical ill health, an adverse external environment, bereavement, ill health of a relative, neglectful children, compulsory retirement and financial difficulties. The data indicated beyond all reasonable doubt that early ascertainment of illness is a highly desirable part of the geriatric service and that assessment must cover the needs of the whole individual.

Though old age is part of normal human development our culture so distorts this phenomenon most of us are afraid to face up to it. An immediate need for the future is a good early education of our young people in successful living with the fullest development of inner resources. In this way future total need may be minimised and ageing development made more meaningful, with more people able to deal effectively with their own problems which arise from within and from without. It is practical to accept the concept that successful ageing is related to the activity of the individual and to its complexity in three areas of life - physical, interpersonal and intellectual, though it is known there are varying types of ageing personalities described as the mature, rocking chair, armoured and angry men and self-haters. Thus it is evident that while late in application the need is urgent for pre- and post-retirement courses and counselling, crafts and hobbies centres, sheltered employment and part-time job placement for retired men and women who wish to work. The Glasgow Retirement Council is an excellent example of such endeavour, but requires to be expanded throughout the country. Should industry and voluntary effort find they cannot meet this demand, Health and Social Work Departments should consider their responsibilities in the matter carefully.

It is inevitable that the continued advances in geriatric medicine will enable more people to live their full life's span and consequently it is to be expected that the numbers in need will increase. Need in terms of multiple disease involving the physical, mental and social spheres of life of the individual. This characteristic complex network of illness makes formidable demands on the knowledge, practical ability and personal security of professional workers, and there are few of us who can attain this high standard. This overflow of responsibility into varied disciplines means that complete success can only be achieved when all workers understand each other's functions and common purpose and integrate their actions. One of the tasks of the Geriatric Units and the Health and Social Work Departments is to bring about this overall integration of effort.

It must be realised that effective resolution of the psycho-social problems of the aged requires a psycho-social casework therapy as outlined, for example, by Hollis[5] in respect of reassurance, guidance, catharsis, reflective consideration of the current person-situation configuration and of the dynamics and development of response patterns or tendencies. Principles of vital importance when working with the aged are acceptance and self-determination and confidentiality with a warmth in the dyadic relationship. The professional worker should feel with and for but not like the old person who is being helped. It is doubtful if many people can learn casework on their own by trial and error, and perhaps the skilled social workers might consider imparting some of their knowledge to those who wish to know. We can only give of our best when time is not at a premium and an important need of the aged is time for conversation and for the observer to listen and understand the real implications of verbal responses and omissions with the appreciation that a person who is ill is very likely to be lonely.

From what has been stated thus far it is evident that the closest liaison must exist between medical and sociological practice and that no elderly person should go without help because they happen to fall in the twilight zone of need between the clear functions of each other. This has relevance to some of the "crisis" situations of old age, for example, bereavement. The need for clarification is possibly more apparent when old age is regarded as a developmental phase of life with its own social and emotional crises and when Caplan's[2] theory is accepted

that intervention is most effective in such situations. The role
of the Social Worker requires to be more positively asserted in
relation to early ascertainment of psycho-social illness, and to
the provision of therapy for the despair and anxiety, the loss of
hope and identity, the loss of self-esteem and disintegration of
integrity, the mental impairment and depression, the frustration
and the irrational desire for independence which are common in
the aged and are frequently associated with social deprivation
and are often seen by the physician in the first instance.

As stated earlier patients with psychological disturbance
are frequently seen at the Rutherglen Centre, the most common
illness being depression. As you know, it is rare for mental
illness to occur in isolation. The environmental, nutritional,
physical and psychological components of an individual are not
discreet and disturbance in any one may involve the others. In
recent work Dr. Judge and I[3] have found that much depressive illness is environmental in nature. The caseworker can literally
save a soul in this form of mental illness which, therefore,
merits amplification. The individuals superficially may give
little evidence of their depression but they are very unhappy.
When the casual agent is reasonably discreet simple listening
can be therapeutic. However, when physical disease is the cause
therapy can be exceedingly difficult and much depends on the
tact, ability and personality of the caseworker. It may be that
depression in old age is to some extent associated with psychic
trauma experienced by them in childhood. Such trauma made them
incapable in adult life of coping with inevitable recurring
losses. Old people so afflicted will discuss their problems and
listen to advice, but they do not possess the inner resources
which would enable them to follow the advice given. This form
of mental illness may benefit from long and intensive caseworker
intervention which has the objective of helping the individual
to understand and resolve fundamental conflicts. It is desirable

to note that depression can, on occasion, precede the appearance of serious organic disease, for example, malignant tumours, endocrine disorders and vitamin deficiencies.

There is no doubt that with the increase in the numbers of general practitioner health centres and the expansion of post-graduate study in geriatrics, and with the attachment of health visitors to general practice and the health visitors screening the elderly population for unmet need which may be physical, mental or social, more will be done for our old people. However, to be as successful as they should be such efforts will require the close involvement of Social Workers with the community geriatric health team composed of the physician in geriatric medicine, the general practitioner, the health visitor and the home nurse. Case conferences, which will be essential to meet the needs of old people, will be invaluable in drawing the various workers together socially. In addition, the clergy have an important role in ascertaining and meeting the needs of the aged.

Where insufficient workers exist to deal with the needs of all old people in an area, then at least an early diagnostic service should be provided for those who are at risk, that is, for those who live alone, the recently bereaved, the recently discharged from hospital, those with defects of movement and those with long-term physical illness.

Until all old people are screened by general practitioner and health visitor for physical disease it would be helpful if social workers, like interested and caring relatives, would be on the look-out for symptoms and signs which suggest the need for general practitioner or health visitor assessment. After all it is a misuse of caseworker time if effort is rendered ineffective by the co-existence of untreated physical disease, for example, a social worker trying to help a socially deprived old lady with poor memory, slowing of reaction time and apathy finds her casework to be unavailing only to be told later that her client suffered from subthyroidism.

A function of a department of geriatric medicine is to maintain the physical, mental and social independence of old people. However, the rehabilitative and reintegrative efforts of geriatric departments will be nullified where related services are deficient, and this has particular relevance for Health and Social Work Departments. There is, of course, a need for more joint assessment units for psychogeriatric patients and for more day hospitals. The community service provisions may be regarded as generally inadequate and this has a bearing on the neglect of the psycho-social needs of the elderly. These provisions are as follows:

(1) Registers of old people are essential and ascertainment of need cannot proceed satisfactorily without accurately compiled registers.

(2) The provision of general practitioner health centres should facilitate the work of Health and Social Work Departments and thereby the work of early ascertainment of illness and of curative therapy. It is desirable that about one in five of general practitioners in such centres and an appropriate proportion of the health visitors receive post-graduate training in geriatric medicine.

(3) One of the important factors in maintaining the independence of an old person is a properly designed house, and local authorities and voluntary effort have responsibilities in this respect. In this way housework is made easer for those who are frail and for those who have to help them. There is a need for sheltered housing with communal social centres under the supervision of wardens. Apart from the usual residential home of the local authority, residential accommodation planned for the special needs of the mentally

frail with some degree of confusion and loss of intellect is required. It is relevant to note that Whitehead[6] is of the opinion that a large number of old people in psychiatric hospitals could be discharged if they had somewhere to go.

(4) Old people need guidance in accident prevention, personal hygiene and nutrition. Drugs should be kept in suitable cabinets and when no longer required returned to the general practitioner or destroyed. The hazard of fire should be reduced to a minimum and sharp pointed and sharp edged utensils should be safely stored. Gas and electrical appliances, wires and plug-points should be inspected in terms of their safe use, while old people should be discouraged from carrying out electrical repairs. The dangers associated with climbing on chairs and up ladders is evident as is the need for adequate lighting of the home and secure floor coverings. In addition, there is the further problem of the prevention of road accidents. Fundamental to the health of the elderly is assessment of their habits, of the form which exercise of the body and the mind takes, of the state of cleanliness of body, clothes and home and the type of clothes worn in relation to the seasons, of the use of leisure time and of the temperance of the individual. In all these matters the health visitors and home nurses are directly involved though, of course, we all have our parts to play in these respects. Furthermore, the home nurses should visit all old people on potent drug therapy to ensure that the general practitioner's orders are being carried out. In this way iatrogenic disease may be minimised. There may be a place for male home nurses to deal with certain types of old men.

Because of the adverse effects of poor dietary habits or nutritional deprivation on physical and mental health and on social behaviour and cognitive status health departments should employ dietitians. The dietitian would, in addition to giving individual advice, be responsible for the education of health visitors, home nurses and others in the nutritional problems of old people. After all a regular daily hot meal is fundamental to the good nutrition of the elderly.

(5) Old people need easily available and adequate services in respect of home helps, meals-on-wheels, chiropody, dental, visual, hearing, physiotherapy, occupational therapy, disability aids, laundry, sitters-in and holiday admission to residential or hospital accommodation for the temporary relief of the load on relatives.

(6) More day centres are required to provide facilities particularly for isolated frail old people. The importance of day centres in terms of nutrition, enhanced interpersonal relationships and broadening of interests cannot be overestimated.

(7) Voluntary effort is an essential part of the community services for the aged and voluntary work should be integrated with the activities of the Health and Social Work Departments. Both departments should provide selected voluntary workers with appropriate training in the problems of the aged, and especially in the basic technique of speaking and listening to the elderly. Day clubs are essential while friendly visiting can be most effective in enabling old people, in need of human warmth and of a feeling that there is someone who is interested in them, to maintain their self-esteem. The Abbeyfield Society shows the excellent provisions which voluntary service can give to the well-being of the aged through suitable accommodation at reasonable rentals, and the voluntary "boarding out" of old people in need merits attention.

(8) Publicity of the statutory and voluntary services which are directed to the elderly is required.

(9) To function properly the community services require adequate transport.

(10) Research is necessary to show more precisely the actual numbers of old people who are in need, and it is worth noting that epidemiological research is an effective way to discover those who are in need. Clearly in the mitigation and prevention of fear, rejection and regression in old age professional workers, and possibly particularly social workers and health visitors, have responsibilities to educate people of all ages, individually and collectively, in the normal aspects of the ageing process, the problems which may be associated with it and in the healthy re-orientation of attitudes and role function.

Rarely in our experience do adult children neglect their aged parents and where this does occur there is likely to be faults on both sides. When such neglect of a parent does exist it is a serious psycho-social problem and the caseworker will find his or her concentration, acceptance and caring taxed to the full. The whole family can be in psychological turmoil as great as is to be found in the problem families of younger age groups. The aged parent by unwarranted accusations and complaints can produce anxiety, guilt and resentment in the minds of the children. It should be noted that while incontinence may be due to organic causes it can also be of psychological origin. Incontinence can be the visible expression of a cry for help and attention or it may be the consequence of an intolerable environmental situation.

Our study of disease and disability inevitably leads us to the problem of death and dying. The needs of the elderly require the possibility to be kept in mind that in our Society anxieties about ageing and dying may lead professional workers and others to neglect old people. Yet it is our duty to lessen the fear of dying and death. An old person who dies in psychological isolation is a reflection on our standard of care, particularly when the worker-dying person relationship can be so rewarding.

Proceeding further it is necessary to realise that feelings of helplessness, hopelessness and despair which have been commented upon earlier can be antecedent to self-destruction, and suicide is a problem of old age. Prevention of suicide is practical for in many cases of attempted suicide there are precursors to the act. The possibility of suicide should therefore be in the minds of those who are involved in meeting the needs of the aged.

As our commitments to the elderly increase those who are in charge of departments should consider the psychological security of their workers. A worker may find difficulty in making a relationship with an elderly person because of unconscious attitudes derived from an early authority figure. The same difficulty may be experienced by a worker who has not come to terms with personal feelings about ageing, disease and death. For such a worker an elderly individual represents a threat, and they are a danger to the health of each other. Furthermore, one must be aware of the possibility of a worker tending to sublimate personal needs in seeking out those who represent mother or father figures.

With the progressive improvements in the care of the aged there should be an expansion in early ascertainment programmes with emphasis on preventive casework. In preventive casework the casework interview is not just a friendly chat though it must contain the elements of friendship, warmth and a desire to help. The interview has a purpose and must therefore be structured and directed, without being authoritative or restrictive. The interviewer has treatment goals in mind. In preventive casework with the elderly, the initial purpose is one of assessment, not only of material circumstances but also of the individual's relationships within the home and in the wider context of his community, and of his adaption to the crises of ageing and retirement. The assessment interview may itself be a therapeutic process, as the individual is offered an opportunity to look back, take stock and sum up. The emotionally mature individual is able to accept himself despite awareness of his shortcomings, and reconcile himself to his past and to his future in spite of frustrations and failures. The alternatives to this integrity is the despair described by Erikson.[4] Despair that time has run out so that it is too late to make good the frustrations of the past and begin anew, and many old people suffer such frustrations. The difference between preventive social work and remedial social work lies in the motivation of the old person. He is not seeking help and does not regard himself as at risk. One must, therefore, establish a meaningful relationship so that he feels the caseworker is interested in and concerned with him.

Having discussed at some length the depressing and optimistic aspects of old age it is apparent that meeting the needs of the elderly is no easy task. The problems can simply be ignored, but this would be a disservice to the aged and an indictment of ourselves. Hope for the aged lies in our giving them a fair share of our working time, our interest and respect.

References

1. Anderson, W.F. and Cowan, N.R. (1955). A consultative health centre for older people. The Rutherglen Experiment. Lancet, ii, 239.
2. Caplan, G. (1961). An approach to community mental health. Tavistock Publications, London.
3. Cowan, N.R. and Judge, T.G. (1968). Undiagnosed social illness in the elderly. Proceedings of the Semmelweis Centenary. Congress of the Hungarian Association of Gerontology, Budapest, p. 50.
4. Erikson, H. (1965). Childhood and society. Penguin Books, London.
5. Hollis, F. (1966). Casework: A psychosocial therapy. Random House, N.Y., p. 72.
6. Whitehead, A. (1970). Hospital management. Geriatric Care Supplement, Sept./Oct., p. 419.

SOCIAL GERONTOLOGY

J.A. HUET

President
International Centre of Social Gerontology,
Paris

Gerontology is becoming a more scientific discipline and more widely recognised yet if we come down to figures, we must agree that there are in the whole world only a few dozen research workers specialising in fundamental gerontological research and less than 300 clinical geriatricians. On the other hand, there are thousands of scientists interested in social gerontology for this is a multidisciplinary science.

Medical and para-medical personnel, sociologists, social workers, psychologists, demographers, statisticians, representatives of churches, economists, financiers and politicians are all concerned in the developments of a science which involves the whole of humanity.

The undernoted five points are of fundamental interest in social gerontology - demography, economics, housing, health and leisure.

DEMOGRAPHY

Anxiety is being created throughout the world by the uncontrolled birth rate, the lowering of infant mortality and the increase in the number of aged people. If the actual rate of reproduction (2% per year) is not diminished, in the year 2,000 the world population, at present 3,700 million will be 7,400 million, i.e. one billion of aged people. In 100 years there will be 25 billion Indians, 20 billion Chinese, 1½ billion Morrocans, 1 billion Egyptians, while seven countries (Asian and Latin American countries) will contain 60 billion inhabitants. These figures mean without a doubt hunger, revolution and wars.

Such an alarming growth of world inhabitants means an outstanding increase in the aged population. Social gerontologists know this and are aware of the catastrophic consequences of lack of understanding of the situation by politicians and send their recommendations to governments demonstrating the efficiency of social gerontology but are doubtful if their opinons will be regarded.

ECONOMICS

A. Ageing of a Nation

The age of a nation is directly related to the number of its aged citizens and the scale of ageing is based on the percentage of people aged 65 and over in the whole population; in industrialised countries the percentage varies from 10 to 20%. In Europe, within the next ten years, the number of aged people will rise to between 18 and 22%, while certain cities, e.g. Berlin in Germany, or Nice in France, there are at present more than 25% of the population aged 65 and over.

Social gerontologists know that such facts lead to <u>recession</u>. With old men at their head industrial plants will keep their old equipment and their old workers. There will be an increase in the "viscosity" of the labour market. With a gerontocracy there is a certain lack of competition, for those who have power are scared at the idea of changing their methods.

In turn recession leads to <u>poverty</u>. When the age equilibrium is endangered by an abnormal increase of old people, the young depart, for the tax burden played by the producers to sustain the non-productive people becomes unbearable. The best workers and the best brains leave the country where life is too difficult for them.

B. <u>National Budgets</u>

Before speaking of the impact of old people on the economic policy of a nation, one should be aware of the figures given in Table 1 by O.C.D.E. (Organisation for Trade and Economic Development) for Europe.

They show (a) the importance of "social expenditure" in the balance of a national budget, and (b) their percentage is high in industrialised countries in expansion, and low in countries where economy is in recession, or in countries where social needs have not yet exploded, e.g., Japan.

They do not show the importance and the cost of the social expenditure specifically alloted to the aged population and the satisfaction of its needs.

These figures show eloquently how and why a national budget can and must be manipulated for the purposes of the economic status of the nation. That is when social gerontologists come in with the evaluation of the needs of aged people.

C. <u>The Necessity of Objective Information</u>

Social gerontology would be unable to give governments sound information without the help of clinical, biological and fundamental research. These disciplines - apparently different - are, in reality, closely linked one to another. They have the same methodology and the same techniques, and must follow the same line to aim at constructive conclusions. There is only one way, i.e. from analysis to synthesis.

D. <u>The "Social Indicators"</u>

There is no valuable social policy without complete knowledge of the numerous "social indicators" which represent the needs of a population.

Table 1

General taxes, social expenses in regard
to the gross national productivity

Countries	1960 General Taxes	1960 Social Expenses	1960 Total	1969 General Taxes	1969 Social Expenses	1969 Total
France	25.95	13.13	39.08	26	18.86	42.86
Germany	27.26	11.82	39.08	29.06	13.06	42.12
Belgium	20.99	7.85	28.84	26.86	10.81	37.67
Italy	20.64	10.54	31.18	21.13	12.72	33.85
Netherlands	24.14	9.37	33.51	27.14	16.58	43.72
Great Britain	26.47	4.15	30.62	36.58	5.94	42.52
Sweden	29.91	5.37	35.48	39	11.28	50.28
U.S.A.	25.56	4.43	29.99	28.32	6.18	34.50
Japan	17.32	3.83	21.15	16.94	4.94	21.88

The needs of aged people represent 10% to 25% of these "social indicators" and it is impossible to ignore them. Social gerontology is the only science - on account of its multidisciplinary components - able to offer a correct approach to these problems, and that is why, more and more, governments and private organisations will encourage its expansion.

HOUSING

One of the most important questions requiring a social policy is housing.

The age of a nation can be judged by the age of its houses. We find old houses containing old people continually exchanging old ideas and youth ready to abandon such deserts. This is what we already see and will see much more if social gerontology does not change the pattern.

A. Housing Problems

Well informed politicians are well aware of the housing needs of their community. They know that if they need the construction of 500,000 apartments per year, they will only get 400,000 built, with each citizen alloted so many square metres. But what politicians ignore is the variation of the requirements according to the age of the inhabitants. Certain districts have an aged population, others have a young population, and the needs of each are quite different. If they are not met, the people will not stay or will be unhappy in homes with facilities badly adapted to their use. This is a situation where social gerontologists should come in, undertake good research and thereafter make sound recommendations.

B. Special Housing for Aged People

Old people do not like to move, they are always frightened at the thought of changing their habits. They prefer to live with their children, even when there are occasional dramatic intergeneration conflicts. Nevertheless, numerous surveys prove that when old people are offered nice homes, well adapted to their needs, with complete security, in a lovely vicinity, not too far out of town, they move there with pleasure. A very good survey on the motivations which determine if old people wish to go into an institution has been made by Butaud. It shows that when they are well informed and sure of what amenities they are going to have, many aged people make up their minds and take a positive decision.

C. Consequences of Ignorance

Insufficient information, or poor, isolated and badly adapted houses or institutions will never attract aged people. Social gerontologists can point out what the consequences are of such conditions. They observe an increase in "urban viscosity", i.e. the people will not move and change apartments, the houses get old and dirty, and even the young people coming from rural areas to find jobs seem to be infected by the same virus of abnormal ageing. At an extreme point, urbanists observe the creation of artificial ghettos with a concentration of the community around two or three shops, and in one or two streets.

D. The Efficiency of Social Gerontology

Fortunately for city councils there are social gerontologists and when they are consulted they are able to appreciate the age and the ageing process of an area and its population. Once the diagnosis has been established they can give sound information and help with the programmes of urbanisation. They know how to change the quality of a population and its potentiality, but this needs the multidisciplinary culture of a skilled social gerontologist.

HEALTH

A. Health Expenditure in a National Budget

Everyone knows the standards established by the World Health Organisation. In the health equipment of a nation, the number of beds alloted to aged people should be 5% for those who are under 65 years, and 55% beds for those above 65, i.e. ten times more. Thus if 15% of a population is aged more than 65, the need in beds for these 15% will be ten times higher than for the rest of the population. It will then cause increased expenses to be recorded in the budget, and an extra tax burden to be paid by the productive part of the population.

When the percentage of aged people exceeds a certain average and is not controlled, the tax burden will become unbearable.

B. Hospitalisation

In similar conditions, the cost of a bed is about the same all over the world. It varies between £8-£10,000 for acute illnesses, and about half that amount for geriatric units where there is less medical and no surgical equipment. Unfortunately, in most European countries, the need for acute beds is such that priority is given to their construction, so there is always a lack of beds for old people (for example, France needs 300,000 beds).

Everybody knows that when winter comes and old people are cold and lonely in their old houses, 49% of acute beds in hospitals are occupied by aged patients.

But how many know that, for the same illness, an adult will occupy a bed during 17 days, while an old patient will stay there for 49 days. This means an expenditure of billions as aged people are often poor and their hospital expenses must be paid by the state.

C. Drug Costs

Aged persons spend 44% more than adults in buying drugs; this is perfectly admissible. What is more difficult to accept is the waste of 60% of these drugs. Old people go to different hospitals or doctors. They are often given different advice and are a chosen prey for quacks. They are always ready to try the "miracle" drug, and their bathroom cupboard is generally full of bottles and boxes of pills. The drug expense for aged people is a constant worry to the social security administrators. Perhaps they could receive efficient advice from social gerontologists.

D. The Triad

All gerontologists know the triad, prevention, treatment and rehabilitation. In this programme where will the social gerontologist be inserted? The solution is clear. The social gerontologist is a multidisciplinary scientist. He is, functionally, a co-ordinator.

To solve the geriatric problem, he will call first on the knowledge of the fundamental research worker. This scientist will give him full information on what is already known and what remains to be done.

He will then go to the demographer to learn what are the demographic trends and what is the short and long-term outlook. What is the age balance in the population, are there some demographic pressures and where are they situated? How can they be handled?

Next he will interview the geriatricians. What is the medical status of the population? What is the epidemiologic equilibrium? What is the health situation of the aged people in hospitals, institutions and homes?

With all this information the social gerontologist will call on the economist who will sum up the needs and evaluate what is required to fulfil them.

All these technical advisers need a "human touch". This should be given by the sociologist, who will himself consult other technicians (psychologists, ecologists, ergonomists, social workers, etc.).

The social gerontologist has now before him the entire pattern of his "human" problem. He has all the material necessary to draw up his final report and to allow him to deliver to the politcal decision-makers valuable information with constructive recommendations.

LEISURE

A. Migrations

Not since the glacial period, when men fled south searching for food, has humanity observed mass migrations like those we see today. Millions and millions of people migrate each year searching for the sun. This creates new sociologic and economic situations. Only 5% to 6% of this huge crowd is made up of aged people. But, as retired people can travel all the year round, their number in Europe alone, can be estimated at 2 to 3 million tourists. Such facts are a matter for business activity, and a rich field of observation for social gerontology.

B. Organisation of Leisure

There is no leisure acceptable and conceivable without freedom of choice. Nevertheless, leisure can be proposed under three models, static for invalids, or people who are unable to travel or even go out of their homes, dynamic for those who are not invalid and can participate in many activities, and kinetic for those who can travel and be active tourists.

This is a major responsibility for the social gerontologist. He must have the necessary knowledge, investigate the needs, appreciate the sociologic, physiologic and economic status of the potential participants, and try to adjust their adaptation to their desires. More and more large cities offer holidays, free of charge, to their old and poor citizens. They must always call on the experience of a social gerontologist.

C. Finances

The Third Age tourism is a new and profitable market. Financiers, tourist agencies, transportation companies are aware of the needs of this new clientele.

Recently T.U.I. (Touristik Union International), one of the most powerful German organisations, has joined with "Transeuropa Reise" (sales by correspondence) and "Darstadt" (chain of supermarkets). They also own Touropa. This means a tourism potentiality of 2,000,000 tourists per year. They estimate at 300,000 the number of aged people and, with social gerontologists, they are preparing special programmes for this special clientele.

This is a new aspect of our civilisation for consumers.

D.   The Role of Social Gerontology

If pure scientists prefer to shut the doors of their ivory tower and refuse to take their place in the moving modern life, it is their right, but for those who have chosen to share the joys and sorrows of their fellow citizens, here is a new opportunity for them to take action. Research in leisure problems is as enriching as research in microcellular changes. The medical, economic and sociologic facts are as fascinating as in any other science, and the reconstitution of this human puzzle needs the skill and the culture of the social gerontologist.

CONCLUSION

It has been demonstrated that social gerontology is a multidisciplinary science and the section of social gerontology was founded in the International Association of Gerontology in London in 1952 by my colleagues and myself. In 1968 a similar group founded the International Centre of Social Gerontology. Such is the progress of this science that in 1952, 40 scientific papers were read in social gerontology at the London meeting, but more than a thousand papers in the same discipline were presented in Kiev in 1972. We, as scientists, must be aware of the desires of humanity and be ready to apply practically new discoveries made. This means that, however it develops, the science of social gerontology must remain multidisciplinary and must be in the vanguard of the whole study of gerontology.

OPERATIONAL RESEARCH AND SOCIAL NEED

MICHAEL HALL

Professor in Geriatric Medicine
University of Southampton

Operational research may be defined as the application of scientific and especially mathematical methods to the study and analysis of complex problems that are not traditionally considered to fall within the field of profitable scientific enquiry. In recent years the Department of Health and Regional Hospital Boards have used the Institute of Operational Research to look at various fields, survey them, measure the current levels of activity and productivity and see how resources may be re-deployed to improve efficiency, e.g. in Wessex (Portsmouth) to see how Gynaecological services may be improved. The fields of study chosen have been relatively circumscribed and to relate operational research to social need and the elderly seems at first sight an impossible task. Nevertheless the first steps to explore this vast uncharted sea are being taken.

Before considering the problem further, the relation between social need and the geriatric patient must be considered. The geriatric patient may be described as an elderly person who has lost the ability to lead an independent unaided existence and consequently needs help to be able to continue to lead a life of quality. His social need is the help which is necessary to enable him to continue to enjoy and live life to his maximum capacity.

Operational research into social need may be either quantitative or qualitative. Obviously quantitative research is easier to do but qualitative research may in fact be more important.

Operational research into the total amount of social provision necessary is essential if the organisation of services to meet social needs and the delivery of those services to the customer is to be rationalised. Each service provided should be organised so that need is met by that service and the customer benefitted; if this does not happen then operational research into the individual service organisation may enable a way to be found to operate the service more effectively. The problem, however, in considering social needs is that these are seldom single; and measurement is difficult, for the effectiveness of a single service is often interdependent upon the provision of other services. Further, it is well recognised that social and medical needs are nearly always inter-related. Consequently if medical needs are efficiently met, the need for social services may be reduced and vice versa. Consequently operational research into any particular social need should take into consideration the effect of that need on other social needs as well as on medical needs. For instance, a very highly organised home care service involving home help, home visitors, a housekeeper service, night sitters and a home nursing service might lessen the need for residential care, hospital beds, meals-on-wheels and many other services. The problem is that nowhere is such a service organised in such a way as to measure its effect upon the other services on which it will impinge. Hence the reason for the word complex in the definition of operational research.

An earlier speaker emphasised that only under controlled conditions can you get any data which you can do anything with (Beckett). This applies particularly to operational research and social need. On the other hand the provision of services cannot await the outcome of academic research. Anyway, many surveys and a considerable weight of sociological and geriatric medical opinion have stressed the importance of many of these social needs. Further, a lot is known about various needs unmet by particular services. Townsend and Wedderburn,[14] for instance, have shown that nearly six times more old people would like to have meals-on-wheels brought than actually receive them. Harris[7] has shown that 62% of recipients of mobile meals wanted extra meals, and included among these were people who already received four meals per week. What has not been estimated is how many of these people would have needed meals-on-wheels if they had been fully and properly assessed in a geriatric unit or what proportion of them would require meals-on-wheels if more luncheon clubs were available and the transport also available to take people to the luncheon clubs, e.g. in Wessex; Bournemouth has a low provision of meals-on-wheels but good luncheon club provision, so that delivery of meals to the elderly is better than in some areas with better meals-on-wheels services. It is, however, essential that agencies providing services are co-ordinated so that those most needing a service get the appropriate dose! If one looks at another service, such as the home help service, it has been shown[8] that this requires quadrupling in some areas. This may well be so, but it is doubtful that in evaluating the service the extent of the other services available in that area was also taken into consideration.

Figure 1 illustrates the provision of some services in England and Wales. A greater provision is necessary and it is worth considering some aspects of the problems which exist in certain selected fields - and in some cases the answers which research indicates.

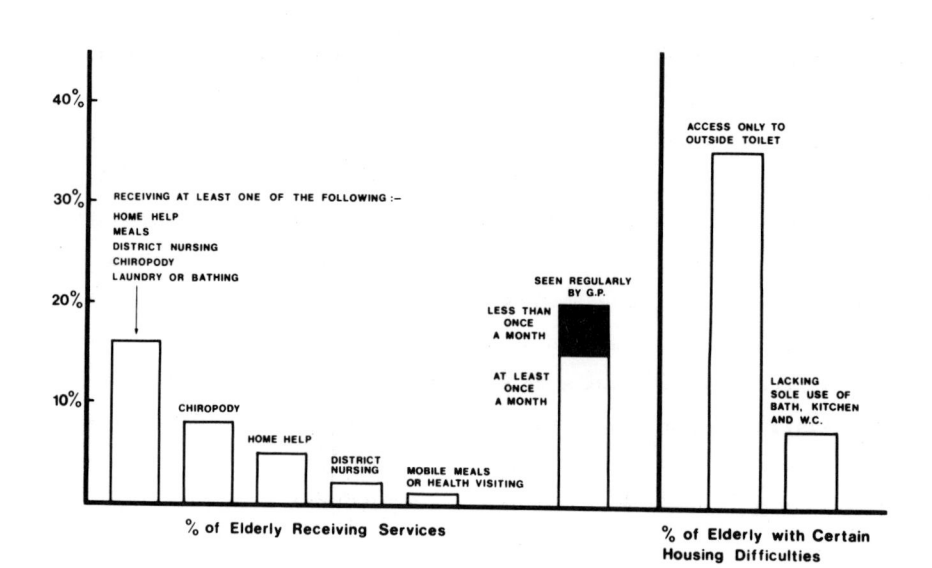

Fig. 1

It is perhaps convenient to review these in relation to the present organisation of the Local Authority's responsibility as shown in Table 1, looking first at education and then housing before considering the provision of more personal services.

There are few physicians in geriatric medicine who would not agree that health education has a vital role to play in reducing the amount of morbidity in the elderly. The need to educate the elderly has already been stressed (Cohen). Both pre- and post retirement education are essential to ensure this. If retirement has been carefully planned, the post retirement period for elderly people can be one of fulfilment and interest. In order to do this however, the essentials must be taken care of; the basic predisposing factors leading to want in old age are as follows:

(a) lack of money;
(b) lack of health;
(c) lack of ability;
(d) lack of conformity.

In order to counteract the first three, pre-retirement education must take place early. Surveys show us that people attending pre-retirement courses know very little about retirement (Table 2). Many of us believe that people benefit from attending pre-retirement courses but how do these really affect the wants and the needs of individuals. Similarly post retirement courses and post retirement education can enable the individual who has planned his retirement to learn new skills and fill his leisure time. It is widely suggested that those who do this are healthier than those who do not. Is this true? By operational research we should be able to discover some of the answers. To do this however, we would need to study the health of the elderly in prescribed areas which have been saturated with pre- and post retirement educational courses and compare these to areas where there was none.

Table 1

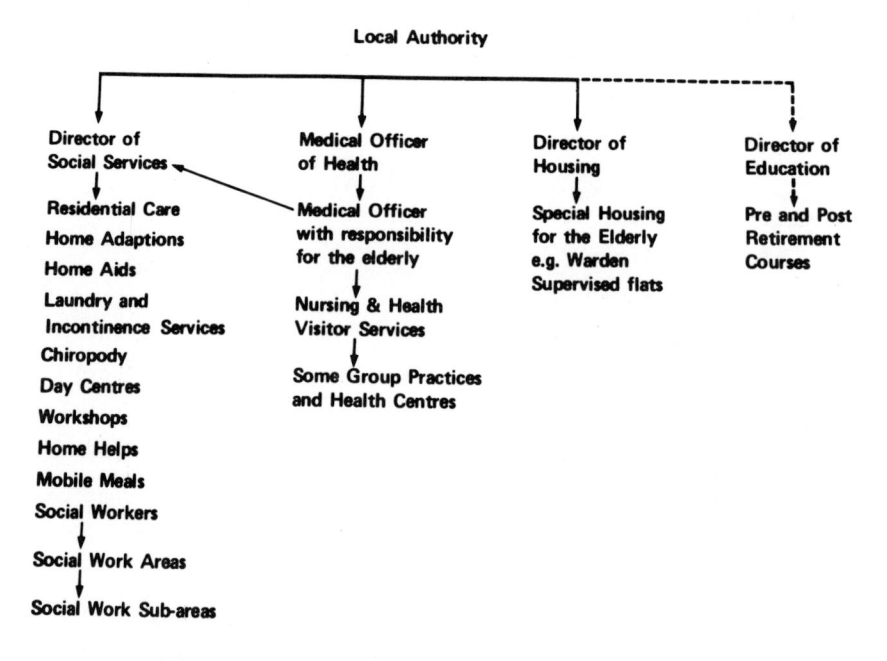

```
                        Local Authority
    ┌───────────────────┬──────────────────┬──────────────────┐
    ▼                   ▼                  ▼                  ▼
Director of         Medical Officer    Director of        Director of
Social Services     of Health          Housing            Education
    │                   │                  │                  │
    ▼                   ▼                  ▼                  ▼
Residential Care    Medical Officer    Special Housing    Pre and Post
Home Adaptions      with responsibility for the Elderly   Retirement
Home Aids           for the elderly    e.g. Warden        Courses
                        │              Supervised flats
Laundry and             ▼
Incontinence Services  Nursing & Health
Chiropody              Visitor Services
Day Centres             │
Workshops               ▼
Home Helps             Some Group Practices
Mobile Meals           and Health Centres
Social Workers
    │
    ▼
Social Work Areas
    │
    ▼
Social Work Sub-areas
```

**TABLE TO SHOW THE PRESENT ORGANISATION OF
LOCAL AUTHORITY SERVICES**

Table 2

Attitudes towards Retirement of 149 men between the Ages of 50 and 55 shows that

105 believed it necessary to go on working in order to keep young;
130 thought the State should provide enough for pensioners to live on;
99 had not considered how they would live on their pension;
93 did not even know what their retirement income would be;
94 had no ideas for the development of new interests;
87 knew nothing about the organisations which might be able to assist them.

It is often said that male mortality in the immediate post retirement period is high and could be related to retirement. Some studies suggest that this is not true and that the health of people in the post retirement period may in fact improve. It is sometimes suggested that retirement brings with it boredom and loneliness and men tend to get depressed, develop illness and die. This suggestion however, is not borne out by the cross national survey[12] in which it was found that healthy men in fact welcomed retirement and did not mind it, whereas those in poor health were the ones who complained about loneliness, missing their workmates, etc. The problem of retirement is for social gerontology to investigate. The effect of alterations of social status, retirement age, lowering of pension age and such like considerations are other factors having a direct bearing on the capability of the individual to meet his social needs. Consequently the effect of any such social alteration needs to be borne in mind inconsidering operational research. This of course particularly relates to the application of operational research - cost benefit analysis and the social gerontologist must be involved.

All physicians in geriatric medicine are I am sure, agreed that the provision of sheltered housing and other suitable housing for the elderly is of vital importance. Surveys[5,17] have suggested that elderly people with medical and psychiatric disability could continue to manage in the community if sheltered housing for the elderly was available. People as they age often become disabled and have to leave their existing homes because these are no longer suitable. If architects and planners were to build houses so that these could be easily adapted for the disabled then this could be avoided. Some enlightened housing authorities, for example, Winchester, have in fact submitted plans for new blocks of flats to specialists in the field of disablement so that flats were designed and built de nova that would be suitable for the disabled to live in should disability arise.[11]

Two recent studies have considered the provision of residential care for the elderly. The first by Jack Hanson[6] was a piece of qualitative operational research specifically designed to study the problem of life in a modern old people's home. He found that the phenomena of block treatment, regimentation, depersonalisation and personal distance all occurred. The study consequently revealed ways in which these phenomena might be avoided. If the lessons learned from this study were applied in other homes, the quality of life of residents could be greatly improved. The second study by Wager[16] was a study which used the framework of cost benefit analysis to compare the working material of the social worker with the working material of the accountant. Basically the study looked at four problems:

(a) The feasibility of domiciliary and residential care as alternatives for the elderly.

(b) The usefulness of an objective assessment of the state of potential clientele for operational purposes.

(d) The establishment of a suitable basis to compare the costs of such different facilities as domiciliary care and residential homes.

(d) The identification of patterns of care that are likely to be less costly without being less effective.

In each case the answer was encouraging. The study is particularly interesting since it raises many problems and provides quite a few answers. For instance, the cost of both the construction and running of residential homes is considered. To provide places for 120 old people would cost probably £16,000 per year extra in three homes of 40 beds, as opposed to two homes of 60 beds, yet the phenomena found by Hanson are more likely to occur in bigger homes. The study also considers the amounts by which the resource costs of residential care exceed those of domiciliary care within various housing circumstances. For instance, for an old person living in "normal" housing with others, the cost differential is around £10 per person per week whereas for those living in sheltered housing the differential is £3 to £4 per person per week. Obviously therefore the provision of sheltered housing with expanded domiciliary care services would seem to offer a better financial bet than the provision of more residential care places. The problem of the provision of both more sheltered housing and more residential care is obviously a considerable one. It has been suggested that perhaps 5.1% of old people need sheltered accommodation. A Government paper[9] suggests that 10.9 special housing units per 1,000 head of population over 65 are necessary. This indicates a five-fold increasing in building. (How practical is this?)

For many years physicians in geriatric medicine have been pointing out the need for much greater provision of local authority services, and this particularly relates to residential care. "Geriatric medicine can now rehabilitate more old people than the social services can reintegrate into society" (Agate[1]). Clark[2,3] has in particular assessed the percentage of disabled ageing patients who can be cared for in residential care, but who for lack of places had to be kept in hospital. As a result of a prospective study he came to the conclusion that 60 hostel beds per annum per 500,000 population were needed after in-patient hospital treatment. This contrasts with the complete absence of any semblance of planning for the required number of places in residential accommodation for the elderly in the future, described by Greta Sumner and Randall Smith[13] in their excellent book 'Planning Local Authority Services for the Elderly'. Vine[15] has estimated that the cost of failure is approximately £3,000 per patient, assuming that the cost of a long-stay hospital bed is £20 per week (the current cost of a long-stay bed in Southampton is £34 per week). There is therefore much evidence to show that planning of sheltered housing and residential care is a subject for close collaboration between Directors of Social Services and housing managers in the local authority field. There is need for many more studies such as that done by Wager[16] for there is no doubt that residential care is expensive.

It is usually agreed that approximately five per cent of the elderly are in some form of residential care, either hospital or local authority provided. It is assumed that there will be 38,300 people over the age of 65 in Southampton in 1981. Consequently we shall require a total of 1,915 places if 5% of these are in residential care or in hospital. In 1977 the local authority will have about 584 places, the hospital will have approximately 330 places - this therefore represents a deficit of 1001 places. The hospital service should be responsible for approximately 500 places which will leave 831 places to be provided by the local authority by 1981. To correct this deficit will require a capital investment of £2,493,000, assuming that present-day costs remain the same and that the land can be provided free. At the present time residential care for the elderly represents an annual revenue cost of £390,000. Since the number of places will need to be increased by almost one and a half times the present number, the annual revenue cost will have to be increased by another £600,000. This would be equal to more than 50% of the total revenue budget of £1,600,000 which is available to the Department of the Director of Social Services at the moment. The importance, therefore, of operational research and cost benefit analysis is clearly demonstrated.

When one considers the services which need to be provided by the Medical Officer of Health (Community Physician) and the Director of Social Services, it is difficult to separate the inter-dependence of services provided by the Directors of Social

Services, Community Physicians and the hospital geriatric services, yet there is an enormous difference in the provision of services for the elderly between regions and areas. Research, however, must be undertaken into the approximate mix or provision of services for the elderly. Surveys conducted from the hospital viewpoint by Droller[4] and Isaacs[10] suggest that community care of the elderly sick is deficient. Droller in his survey suggests that 25% of his sample could have been cared for at home if necessary services had been available. He regards the most important of these services to be as follows:

1. Geriatric Advisory Clinic;
2. Home Help;
3. Alternative housing;
4. District Nurse;
5. Regular visiting;
6. Soiled laundry service;
7. Chiropody;
8. Physiotherapy;
9. Meals-on-wheels;

whereas Isaacs suggests that in addition to this wider range of social services we must also improve hospital services:

1. improve hospital turnover;
2. promote earlier case finding;
3. expand day and outpatient care;
4. provide wider range of social services;
5. provide intermittent relief.

Few would disagree with these observations. The problem is how may this be most effectively done.

There are plenty of people both in the field and in the hospital service to be able to deal with the problems of the elderly, but their efforts must be better co-ordinated. This could be done if social work areas, or in some cases sub-areas, were taken as the basic units for the delivery of services. Operational research would then be possible within the area or sub-area and these could be compared to one another. Since the mix of services available would vary, it would be possible to compare the effectiveness of various "mixes" in maintaining independence or lessening dependence. Only by so organising and structuring the pattern of the care provided will we be able to measure its effect and provide adequate and rational services designed to meet the social needs of the elderly.

References

1. Agate, J. (1970). The Fifth Social Service. Fabian Society.
2. Clark, A.N.G. (1963). Residential care of the disabled aged. Geront. clin., $\underline{5}$, 38.
3. Clark, A.N.G. (1964). Discharge failure in hospital practice. Geront. clin., $\underline{6}$, 224.
4. Droller, H. (1969). Does community care really reach the elderly sick? Geront. clin., $\underline{11}$, 169.
5. Green, M. and Lodge, B. (1965). The needs of the elderly in the hospitals and welfare homes of Barrow in Furness. Geront. clin., $\underline{7}$, 20.
6. Hanson, J. (1972). Residential care observed. Age concern and Nat. Inst. Social Work Training.
7. Harris, A. (1960). Meals-on-wheels for old people. Nat. Corpn. for the Care of Old People.
8. Harris, A. (1968). Social welfare for the elderly. Vol. 1. H.M.S.O.
9. Health and Welfare: the development of community care. (1966) Cmnd 3022, H.M.S.O.
10. Isaacs, B. (1971). Studies of illness and death in the elderly. Scottish Home and Health Department.
11. Russell Grant, W. Personal Communication, 1971.
12. Sharnas, E., Townsend, P., Wedderburn, D., Friis, H., Milhøj, P. and Stehouwer, J. (1968). Old people in three industrial societies. Routledge and Kegan Paul.
13. Sumner, G. and Smith, R. (1969). Planning local authority services for the Elderly. George Allen and Unwin.
14. Townsend, P. and Wedderburn, D. (1965). The aged in the welfare state. Bell.
15. Vine, S.M. (1969). Analaysis and cost of failure. Geront. clin., $\underline{11}$, 13.
16. Wager, R. (1972). Care of the elderly. Inst. of Municipal Treasurers and Accountants.
17. Woodside, M. (1965). Hospital and community experience of 150 psychiatric patients. Geront. clin., $\underline{7}$, 286.

THE WAY AHEAD

WILLIAM FERGUSON ANDERSON

Professor of Geriatric Medicine
University of Glasgow

Area Service
In regard to the future of geriatric medicine, the important point to stress is that as a speciality geriatric medicine has worked. In those countries which have adopted the principle whereby a physician becomes particularly interested in older people and is given adequate supporting staff, secretarial assistance, and the hospital facilities which he needs, immense improvement in the care of older people has occurred.

Older people require a wide spectrum of service. This ranges from housing of modern type to continuing treatment hospital accommodation, and includes the need for many varieties of domiciliary services. With increasing age the elderly are vulnerable to failing physical health and deterioration of mental health perhaps as a result of bereavement, fear, retirement and loss of status in the community.

Methodology
Organisation of a geriatric service depends on a basic methodology with the endeavour to keep the older person happy

and healthy in his own home. In order to do this, <u>ascertainment</u> i.e. the seeking out of the older person in his own home is necessary to discover illness. The self-reporting of symptoms to the doctor is not a satisfactory way of finding out disease early in the upper age ranges. <u>Preventative measures</u> can then be commenced to try to contain the illness found and stop further deterioration. Such individuals discovered to be failing in health in the community must be <u>supervised</u> for life so that they can remain where they desire to be in their own homes. Once illness has occurred, accurate <u>assessment</u>, correct <u>diagnosis</u> or list of diagnoses and appropriate <u>therapy</u> must be undertaken and continued <u>follow-up</u> of the old person organised. It may be essential to admit the older person to an acute medical or surgical unit or a geriatric unit because of ill health, for treatment or diagnosis, and the factors associated with illness in older people, such as physical disease, mental ill health and social deprivation must be kept in mind.

In the organisation of a geriatric service one primary unit in cities is the health centre, or if this is not acceptable, the local service can be based on the group practice.

The Health Centre

Ideally in geriatric work, general practitioners work in groups of five to eight in a health centre, and serve a population of 20,000-30,000 people. In such a community there will be approximately 2,000-3,000 people 65 years and over.

At the general practitioner health centre all members of the health team can meet together and the domiciliary, community and hospital services can be linked for the benefit of the older individual. Specialists may visit the health centre from the hospital, including the psychiatrist and physician in geriatric medicine. The district nursing, health visitor and social services will be co-ordinated there, meeting with representatives of voluntary organisations. Ministers of Religion will look in regularly and perhaps eventually one day the payment of pensions will also be organised from a health centre. The old person or their relatives should only require to make enquiries from one centre to obtain the help or assistance which they require. In an area geriatric service the physician in geriatric medicine, visiting the health centre regularly, will organise three main services:

(1) an ascertainment service in co-operation with the general practitioners and the health visitors;

(2) an out-patient session to help his general practitioner colleagues; and

(3) will encourage and stimulate the local general practitioners in the care of their elderly patients.

The health visitor will visit every person considered to be a risk, for example, those 70 years and over in the area served by the health centre, using a validated proforma providing essential information about the physical, mental and social condition of the older person, and will report to the older individual's own general practitioner. He will liaise with the consultant in geriatric medicine and will examine those few individuals found by the health visitor to require medical examination; this will not be a large number of people. Any problem of housing or requirement of social service will be referred to the representative of the Director of Social Service. The endeavour will be to organise a preventive service to try and maintain the health of older people in the community.

An out-patient session at the health centre would be organised and old people would be seen by the physician in geriatric medicine at the request of their own general practitioner.

The district nurse and health visitor from the community nursing team and the general practitioners would be stimulated by the visit of the geriatric physician.

Chiropody, occupational therapy, domiciliary physiotherapy, alteration to house, admission of older people to allow relatives to go on holiday, or better supply of housekeepers to the older person's own home - information about these services should be available from the health centre. The home help service would be organised at health centre level and a dietitian would visit the health centre to give advice to all those working in the patient's home, making sure that the food provided for the meals-on-wheels service, based on the health centre, were appropriate for the elderly.

The Area Geriatric Service

The components of this are: hospital beds, acute for intensive care; the geriatric unit for illness requiring the special facilities of such a unit; beds in the mental hospital for those requiring the specialised services of the psychiatrist; and a small psychogeriatric unit for those elderly patients unacceptable to the psychiatrist, the physician in geriatric medicine or the director of social service. By having a similar area of responsibility for the mental hospital, the acute beds and the geriatric unit agreement between the general physicians, physicians in geriatric medicine and the psychiatrists would be reached.

The hospital service would also provide a day hospital and out-patient facilities and attached to each teaching and district hospital would be continuing treatment hospital units, possibly in two locations; one in the area of the teaching hospital and other smaller units of continuing treatment beds in the areas served by the health centres. It is important, both in patients with gross physical disease and those with continuing mental disability that they should not be accommodated in large units, and that if the treatment has to go on until the patient dies, these units should be as near the locality from which the patient comes as possible.

The other essential constituents of the area geriatric service are homes for the physically frail, homes for the mentally frail, and a correct proportion of protected housing. These are apart from any specialised dwelling built for old people.

In an area of around 200,000 inhabitants there should be an assessment unit in the district or teaching hospital of approximately 50 beds, with a geographically separate area for mentally disturbed people. Continuing treatment hospital beds should be available to bring the total for the 200,000 inhabitants to about 400 beds.

The geriatric services would be under the control of three physicians in geriatric medicine who would have a defined area with a definite population. The geriatric assessment unit would be in the principal hospital, either teaching or district, for the area and in that hospital, as well as acute beds, there would be beds for the psychiatrist, so that all services in the future would be co-ordinated from one hospital. The out-patient department and day hospital for the elderly would also be situated there. Unless there are sufficient hospital beds to avoid a waiting list for older individuals, the geriatric service cannot function properly. The acute assessment unit would be used to take patients who were ill and who required geriatric treatment, from their own homes, with emphasis placed on the need for accurate early diagnosis. The unit should be used not only for elderly individuals whose physical, mental or social health has considerably disintegrated but also for relatively fit older people who were unwell with an unknown illness. The need for accurate diagnosis is predominant and this must be constantly stressed in the teaching of the medical student.

Sufficient beds should be available in the continuing treatment hospital units to ensure that older people in acute wards in other sectors of the hospital should not occupy expensive beds to the disadvantage of the hospital service. Approximately 18 beds per 1,000 of those aged 65 years and over gives a proper estimate in most areas of the number of geriatric beds, but this figure will vary from place to place and the service cannot perform its function without a satisfactory number of beds.

Homes for Physically and Mentally Frail

In association with the district or teaching hospital there should be homes for the physically and mentally frail; there is an outstanding demand for place in such homes. The number of beds in specialised homes for the physically frail old people, should be around 2.5 places per 1,000 of the population. In future it will be essential to have homes for the mentally frail for individuals who have passed through the diagnostic net of the physician in geriatric medicine and the psychiatrist, and for whom no further hospitalisation is considered necessary. Many of these individuals will be continuing on tranquilising medicine but will be biddable. It is recommended that there is need for around five places in such specialised homes for every 1,000 people 65 years and over and no one should be admitted to such a home without a comprehensive examination by a psychiatrist and/or a physician in geriatric medicine. Admission to a geriatric unit or a mental hospital may be required before a correct diagnosis can be made. Regular visits by the physician in geriatric medicine should be made to homes for the physically frail and it is recommended that the psychiatrist should also be visiting from time to time the homes for the mentally frail.

It is difficult to estimate the number of beds which will in the future be required in psychiatric accommodation but from previous experience it can be dogmatically recorded that shortage of beds in one part of a comprehensive service, produces overloading and breakdown in other sectors.

Sheltered Housing

These homes for the physically frail and the mentally frail should not be regarded as end points in a system. Older people admitted to such places may with care and attention, and appropriate therapy, improve so much that they can advance to proected or sheltered housing. This type of housing has taken over from the traditional old person's home and with a 24-hour supervision by a warden, can give the old person freedom of action, ability to communicate in a friendly way with neighbours and yet be protected by someone being on call all the time. There is great need for rapid expansion of such housing and it is recommended that 50 sheltered houses be provided for every 1,000 people 65 years and over.

Domiciliary Services

Domiciliary services of all varieties will require to be extended and the use of specially trained home helps for mentally confused individuals and of home helps acting as night sitters-in undoubtedly will become more widespread. The use of trained housekeepers to allow relatives looking after the elderly to obtain a holiday is worth consideration. This method avoids the upset of physical or mental health of the elderly person transferred to hospital for this purpose.

In addition to the services mentioned above, laundry for the incontinent, provision of specialised equipment on loan and adaption of house, where required, to suit disabled people are all required.

Staffing

In the geriatric unit itself there will be a team consisting of physicians in geriatric medicine, supporting medical staff, specially trained nurses, physiotherapists, occupational therapists, chiropodists, speech therapists, and secretarial assistants and, as detailed above, the domiciliary team based on the health centre will consist of district nurse, health visitor, physiotherapist, occupational therapist, chiropodist, social worker and voluntary worker.

Co-ordination

Co-ordination between the health centre and the hospital would be accomplished by the physician in geriatric medicine coming from the hospital to the health centre and by the social worker in the hospital being in contact with the social worker in the health centre. The flow-through geriatric units in the teaching or district hospital depends on the provision of adequately trained personnel, proper equipment and first-class amenity and cannot be accomplished without continuing treatment hospital accommodation, day hospital and day centre facilities. Linked to this must be adequate follow-up services based on the health centre with appropriate accommodation for physically and mentally frail older people and a wide range of domiciliary services.

Pre-Admission Assessment Visit

Many physicians in charge of geriatric units have found great advantage in paying an assessment visit to the ill old person's home before admission following the request by the general practitioner for assistance. This procedure ensures that the hospital doctor has knowledge of the patient's home circumstances and the presence or absence of caring relatives, and provides an excellent opportunity for informing the patient of his future plans. The time that elapses between the visit of the specialist and admission to hospital can be utilised to build up the mental health of the elderly individual by explaining repeatedly that she is coming into hospital to get well. After discharge from the appropriate hospital it is advisable to continue to keep the elderly person under supervision by a visit from a health visitor or district nurse.

Pre-Retirement Training

Training for retirement is now essential and there is an increasing tendency for technical colleges to run classes just before or after lunch, combined with lunch. This has attracted the attention of many older people and these courses have proved of great value.

Re-training for useful employment will be desired by a certain number of the elderly and re-employment bureaux, where started, have been successful. The demand for extra-mural classes and training for elderly individuals will increase and many people will want the provision of such classes as they grow old.

It is obvious that the mental health of the older individual must be looked at with much greater care and work such as that of Newman's on incontinence, studied afresh, and consideration given to the depression and feeling of impending dissolution, which accompanies admission to hospital.

Enough information is now available to provide an area geriatric service for old people. The type of service required for most elderly people is now known and the provision of a varied spectrum of such services will meet the needs of most people. Information is still woefully lacking on now to re-house older people successfully and while much work has been done on this subject, more study is needed. At this time, however, enough information is in our possession to provide, if we so desire, an area geriatric service which will meet the requirements of the great majority of fit, frail and ill older people.

The last ten years have seen an immense and rapid expansion of academic interest in geriatric medicine. In the United Kingdom the first chair in this subject was founded in 1965 and there are now seven such professors. To those who teach, the outstanding interest of young people in the elderly has been abundantly demonstrated; this augurs well for the future.

SUBJECT INDEX

Abbeyfield Society, 277
Abnormal tongue, 253
Accident prevention, 276
Acromegaly, 165
Adaption of house, 313
Adriamycin, 188
Advances in psychiatry, 43
Advances in psychology, 43
Affective disorders, 96
Age and food intakes, 248
Age changes in mental function, 108, 109
Ageing, 166
Ageing of a nation, 284
Ageing process, 43
Aggression, 69
Alkaline phosphatase, 259
Alternative housing, 304
Amantadine, 172, 181
Amitriptyline, 59
Ampulla of Vater, 192
Amyloidosis, 215, 222
Angular stomatitis, 253, 254
Anoxaemia, cerebral, 52
Anticonvulsants, 163
Anti-depressants, 59, 71
Anti-diuretic hormone, 164
Anti-psychotics, 55
Aortic sclerosis, 214
Aortic valve stenosis, 214
Area geriatric service, 310
Arousal, autonomic, 54
Arousal effect, 174

Arterial syndrome, 141
Arteriosclerotic Parkinsonism, 171
Ascertainment, 308, 309
Ascorbic acid, 252
Assessment by health visitor, 274
Assessment, psychiatric, 79
Assessment unit, 311
Assessment visit, 314
Asthma, 206
At risk groups, 78
Atrophic gastritis, 192
Attitude to age, 9
Autonomic arousal, 54
Auxiliary, nursing, 24

Bacterial endocarditis, 215
Bacteruria, 124
Barium swallow, 192
Basal metabolic rate, 251
Beclamethasone aerosol, 217
Beef red tongue, 253
Behavioural disturbance, 50
"Benvil", 54
Bereavement, 100, 272
Beri-Beri, 239
Biliary disease, 259
Biochemical factors, 70
"Biogastrone", 193
Bladder, 123
Block treatment, 301
Bone rarefaction, 121
Bowel, 123

SUBJECT INDEX

Bradykinesia, 173
Brain failure, 110
Brain metabolism, 137
Bronchial asthma, 206
Bronchial carcinoma, 205
Busulphan, 189
Butyrophenones, 56

Carbenoxolone sodium, 193
Carbimazole, 160
Carbohydrate, 233, 235
Calcitonin, 164
Calcium, 259
Calcium metabolism, 161
Calorie requirements, 233, 234
Carcinoma, bronchial, 205
Carcinoma of colon, 193
Carcinoma, gastric, 192
Cardiac amyloidosis, 215
Cardiac disease, 213
Cardiac efficiency, 136
Cardiac failure, 178
Cardiology, 213
Cardiomyopathy, 222
Carotene, 235
Carotid insufficiency, 137
Casework, 279
Cell fall out, 137
Cerebellar ataxia, 158
Cerebral anoxaemia, 52
Cerebral blood flow, 64, 110, 111
Cerebral vasodilators, 110

Cerebrovascular insufficiency, 137
"Ceteprin", 128
Changes in mental function, 174
Chiropodist, 6
Chiropody, 277, 310, 304
Chlorambucil, 180
Chlordiazepoxide, 53
Chlorpromazine, 52, 56, 159
Chronic brain syndrome, 124
Chronic bronchitis, 204
Chronic myeloid leukaemia, 186
Chronic sick nursing, 22
Chronic respiratory disease, 203
Cine film, 14
Circadian rhythm, 155
Clinical features of depression, 71
Clinico-pathological correlation, 120
Collateral cerebral circulation, 136
Colon, carcinoma of, 193
Colon, diverticular disease of, 195
Colonoscope, 193
Coloured matrices, 82, 90
Community mental health, 91
Community physician, 303
Community problems, 43
Community surveys, 77
Complex drug regimes, 149
Concern, public, 35
Conditioned nutritional disease, 232

SUBJECT INDEX

Confusion, 51, 158
Constipation, 72, 129
Continuing treatment unit, 310
Control, postural, 5
Controlled education programme, 21
Corneal calcification, 163
Corticosteroids, in asthma, 206
"Cosaldon", 112
Craft centres, 271
Crichton behavioural rating, 82, 174
Crichton vocabulary, 82
Crises, 272
Croakiness, 158
Cross-national survey, 300
Cryptic disseminated tuberculosis, 208
Customer benefit, 294
Cyclandelate, 112
"Cyclospasmol", 112
Cyclophosphamide, 187, 189
Cytosine arabinoside, 187

Dancing bear syndrome, 56
Daunorubicin, 186
Day centres, 277
Day clubs, 277
Day hospital, 310
Deafness, 158
Death and dying, 278, 279
Death and vitamin C, 258
Death from gastric ulcer, 193
Deficient collagen, 162

Degenerative calcification, 215
Degenerative calcific valve disease, 214
Deglycyrrhizinized liquorice, 193
Dementia, 73, 82, 96, 107, 138, 139, 160, 256
Demography, 283
Dentist, 277
Dentition, 262
Dentures, 241, 253
Depersonalisation, 301
Depression, 44, 50, 67, 68, 100, 107, 174, 273
Depression, clinical features, 71
Depression, management, 72
Depression, prevention, 73
Depression, reactive, 69
Diagnosis, 308
Diagnosis of malnutrition, 248
Diazepam, 52, 53
Dichloralphenazone, 55
Dietary deficiencies, 73
Dietitian, 310
Digoxin toxicity, 222
Director of Social Work, 309
Disability aids, 277
"Disipal", 58, 178
Disodium cromoglygate, 207
District nurse, 304
Disturbed awareness of self and space, 141
Diverticulae, duodenal, 194
Diverticular disease of colon, 195

SUBJECT INDEX

Domiciliary care, 301
"Doriden", 232
Drop attacks, 140
Drug absorption, 150
Drug activity, 150
Drug administration, 149
Drug competition, 151
Drug costs, 289
Drug excretion, 151
Drug holidays, 58
Drug reactions, 120
Drug therapy, 149
Drug toxicity, 111
Drugs, psycho-active, 47
Duodenal diverticulae, 194
Duodenal tumours, 192
Duodenal ulceration, 192
Duodenitis, 192
Dyskynesia, 178
Dysphagia, 192
Dystonia, drug induced, 54
Dysuria, 123

Early diagnosis, 45
Early waking, 71
E.C.G., 220
E.C.G. monitoring, 181
Economics, 284
E.C.T., 63
Education, 3, 4
Education, nurse, 19
Efficiency of social gerontology, 288

Emepronium bromide, 128
Emotional disturbance, 50
Endocarditis, 215, 216
Endocrinology, 153
Energy expenditure, 251
Enrolled nurse, 22
Environment, 43
Environment and mental health, 95
Environmental stress, 99
Epidemiology of incontinence, 123
Equipment, 11
Equipment loan, 313
Erythrocyte glutathione reductase, 254
Essential tremor, 172
Ethambutol, 209
Exercise tolerance, 142
Experimental variables, 44
External sphincter, 126

Faecal impaction, 129
Faecal incontinence, 123, 129
Faradism, 127
Features of Parkinsonism, 171
Feedback information, 18
"Fentazin", 56
FEV, 199
Fever, 5
Fibre-optic endoscopy, 191
Finance, 291
Five-hydroxoindole-acetic acid, 71
Fluoride, 162
Fluphenazine, 56

SUBJECT INDEX

Fluphenazone decanoate, 58
Fluphenazine enathate, 58
Folic acid, 239, 240, 255, 256
Follow-up, 73, 91, 308
Food-behaviour patterns, 228, 232
Food expenditure, 233, 235
Food intakes and age, 233, 248
Food selection, 228
Food supplements, 264
Forced expiratory volume, 199
Forced vital capacity, 199
Fractures, 161, 207, 260
Frequency of micturition, 72
Functional illness, 50
FVC, 199

Gairdner, Dr. W., 39
Gastric carcinoma, 192
Gastric ulcer, death from, 193
Gastric ulceration, 193
Gastroenterology, 191
Generic social work, 33
Genetic factors, 96
Geriatric Advisory Clinic, 304
Geriatric Medicine, 3, 307
Geriatric Neurology, 171
Geriatrics, Preventative, 5
Gerontology, 283
Glasgow Retirement Council, 271
Glasgow surveys, 78
Glutethamide, 232
Gonadotrophins, 154
Growth hormone, 165

Hallucinations, 51
Haloperidal, 52, 57
Health centre, 308
Health expenditure, 288
Health visitor, 78, 274, 309
Hearing aids, 277
Heart block, 222
Heart disease, 213
Hemiblock, 217
Hereditary factors, 98
"Hexopal", 112
Hexyl theobromine, 112
High residue diet, 196
Hobbies centres, 271
Holiday admission, 277
Home helps, 277, 304, 310, 313
Hormones, 153
Hospital, acute, 22
Hospital, long-stay, 22
Hospital service, 303
Hospitalisation, 289
Housebound, 259
Houses for the frail, 312
Housing, 287
Housing problems, 287
Housing, unsuitable, 37
Hypercalcaemia, 163
Hypercalciuria, 161
Hypertensive heart disease, 220
Hypochondriacal complaints, 72
Hypothalamic pituitary area, 154
Hypothalamic pituitary function, 155

SUBJECT INDEX

Hypothermia, 120, 159, 254, 258
Hypothyroidism, 155, 157
Hyroxyproline, 257

Iatrogenic hypothyroidism, 157
Iceberg phenomenon, 270
Idiopathic parkinsonism, 172
Ignorance, 288
Imipramine, 59
Immunotherapy, 187
Improving nutrition, 263
Incontinence, 123, 124
Incontinence chart, 129
Incontinence, faecal, 123, 129
Incontinence, urinary, 123, 126
"Inderal", 54
Indwelling catheters, 129
Inosital nicotinate, 112
"Intal", 207
"Integrin", 57
Intellectual performance, 64
Internal sphincter, 126
Intestinal ischaemia, 195
Intoxication, 48
Intra-cardiac conduction, 216
Intracranial vessels, 136
Involutional melancholy, 68
Iron, 241
Ischaemia heart disease, 218, 220
Ischaemia modifying factors, 137

Isolation, 68, 101, 262, 270
Isoniazid, 209
Isoprenaline, 222

Jejunal biopsy, 195

L-asparginase, 187, 188
L-thyroxine, 156
L-tri-iodo-thyronine, 156
"Largactil", 52, 56, 159
Laundry, 277, 313
Lean body mass, 251
Lecture room facilities, 11
Left anterior hemiblock, 217
Leisure, 291
"Lentizol", 60
Leucocyte ascorbic acid, 252, 256, 257
Leukaemia, 185, 186, 187
Leukaemia deaths, 185
Levodopa, 172
Levodopa, side effects, 172
"Librium", 53
Lithium, 61
Liver disease, 259
Longitudinal study, 91
Loneliness, 68, 69, 73, 262
Longmore disability score, 113, 114
Low dosage, 49
"Lucidril", 112
Luncheon club, 295
Lung volume, 203

SUBJECT INDEX

Magenta tongue, 253
Magnesium, 242
Malabsorption, 162, 194, 259
Male mortality, 300
Malnutrition, 247, 248
Management of depression, 72
Mania, 50
Mature personality, 98
Meclofenoxate, 112
Meals-on-wheels, 277, 295, 304, 310
Meat, 241
Mebeverine, 196
Medical needs, 247
Medicine, Geriatric, 3
Megaloblastic anaemia, 255
"Mellerill", 55, 56, 58
Memory, drugs and, 107
Memory tests, 82
Mental barriers, 141
Mental health, 67
Mental illness, 270
Mental state, 95
Mentally impaired at home, 229
Meprobamate, 54
Metabolic brain disease, 111
Methodology, 307
Methotrexate, 187
Methylcellylose, 196
Methyl dopa, 71
Migrations, 291
Milieu interieur, 151
Milk, 236, 238

"Miltown", 54
Mitral valve, 214
"Modicate", 58, 59
Modicate clinics, 58
"Moditen", 56
"Mogadon", 55
Monoamine oxidase inhibitors, 60, 71
Monoamine oxidase levels, 71
Mood, 70
Mood change, 51
Motivation, 142
Motor deficit, 142
Mucosal change, intestinal, 195
Multifactorial concept, 78
Multiple pathology, 5, 67
Myocardial insufficiency, 213

Naftidrofuryl, 112
"Nardil", 60
National budgets, 285, 288
Needs of nurses, 21
Neoplasm, 164
"Neulactil", 57
Neuroses, 50
Nicotinic acid, 238, 253
Night sitters, 313
Nightingale, Florence, 21, 23
Nitrazepam, 55
Nocturia, 72, 124
Noradrenaline, 71
Nurse, 6
Nurse, education, 19

SUBJECT INDEX

Nurse, enrolled, 22
Nurses, pupil, 21
Nursing auxiliary, 24
Nursing officer, 25
Nutrition, 231
Nutritional allowances, 232
Nutritional disease, 44
Nutritional guidance, 276
Nutritional requirements, 231
Nutritional surveys, 247

Objective information in sociology, 285
Occult alimentary blood, 192
Occupational therapy, 6, 277
Oestrogens in incontinence, 127
Old people's home, 301
Operational research, 121, 293
Organ scanning, 191
Organic brain changes, 97
Organic illness, 50
Organisation, 307
Orphenadrine, 58, 178
Orthostatic hypotension, 174
Osteomalacia, 163, 260
Osteoporosis, 161
Outpatient session, 309, 311
Overdosage, 48
Oxazepam, 53
Oxpertine, 57

PAS, 209
P.B.I., 156

Pacemaker, 222
Pads and appliances, 128
Paget's disease, 164
Pain, 5
Paranoid states, 50
Para-medical personnel, 283
Parkinsonism, 171
Parkinsonism, arteriorsclerotic, 171
Parkinsonism, idiopathic, 171
Partial gastrectomy, 193
Pathology, multiple, 5
Pellagra, 238
Pelvic floor exercises, 127
Perception, 227
Pericolic abscess, 196
Pericyazine, 57
Peritonitis, 196
Perphenazine, 56
Personal hygiene, 276
Personality, 97, 98
Personality inventory, 82
Personality, mature, 98
Phenelzine, 60
Phenothiazines, 56
Phosphorus, 259
Photo-toxicity, 56
Physical disease, 70, 273
Physical state, 51
Physiological studies, 120
Physiotherapy, 6, 277, 304
Polypharmacy, 152
Post-basic course, 22

SUBJECT INDEX

Post-retirement courses, 271
Postural control, 5, 143
Postural imbalance, 138
Potassium, 241
Potassium depletion, 121
Poverty, 37, 284
Poverty of reserve, 138
Practolol, 161
"Praxilene", 112
Prednisone, 186, 207
Pre-retirement clinics, 100
Pre-retirement courses, 271, 297, 315
Prevalence of Parkinsonism, 172
Preventative geriatrics, 5, 269
Preventative measures, 308
Preventive service, 309
Prevention, 290
Prevention of accidents, 276
Prevention of depression, 73
Prevention of vitamin deficiencies, 261
Primary hypothyroidism, 157
Primary nutritional disease, 232
Principals of therapeutics, 49
Principal sources of nutrients 232, 233, 236
Professional specialisation, 34
Profile of patient liable to develop depression, 74
Programme, teaching, 11

Prolapse of urethral mucosa, 126
Propranalol, 54
Prostaglandins, 154
Protein, 232, 233
Psychiatric assessment, 79
Psychiatric symptom sign inventory, 82
Psychiatrist, 311
Psychiatry, advances in, 43
Psycho-active drugs, 47
Psycho-geriatric service, 102
Psycho-geriatric unit, 310
Psychometric tests, 79
Psychology, advances in, 43
Psycho-social case work, 272
Public concern, 35
Pulmonary tuberculosis, 204, 208
Pulmonary ventilation and perfusion, 200
Pupil nurses, 21
Pupil nurse training, 27

Radio-immuno assays, 153, 156
Radiological indices, 161
Radiotherapy for bronchial carcinoma, 205
Random samples, 79, 218, 248
Reactive depression, 69
Recession, 284
Recreation, 73
Regional blood flow, 138
Regimentation, 301
Registers of elderly, 275
Regular visiting, 304

SUBJECT INDEX

Reintegration, 302
Rejection, 101
Rejection syndrome, 101
Relatives, 10
Renal disease, 163
Research, 119
Research design, 44
Reserpine, 71
Residential care, 301, 303
Respiratory disease, 199
Restlessness, 51
Retirement, 4, 99, 100
Retirement councils, 271
Retirement counselling, 73
Retrobulbar neuritis, 209
Retrograde cholangiography, 192
Riboflavine, 236, 253, 254
Rifampicin, 209, 210
Right bundle branch block, 217

Scurvy, 256
Secondary hypothyroidism, 157
Secondary nutritional disease, 232
Senescence, 86, 96
Senile cardiac failure, 213
Senile psychosis, 98
Senior Nursing Officer, 25
Sensory deficit, 142
"Serenid-D", 53
"Serenace", 52, 57
Services for the Elderly, 295
Sheet haemorrhages, 256

Sheltered employment, 271, 315
Sheltered environment, 102
Sheltered housing, 275, 300, 313
Side effects, levodopa, 172, 179
Sitters-in, 277
Skin-fold thickness, 235
Social deprivation, 101
Social factors, 68
Social gerontology, 283
Social indicators, 285
Social isolation, 270
Social needs, 247, 305
Social problems, 43
Social Worker, 6, 33
Sociologists, 283
Soiled laundry services, 304
Special homes for mentally frail, 102
Special housing, 287
Specialist training, 5
Speech therapist, 6
Staff-patient ratios, 20
Status epilepticus, 53
"Stelazine", 56, 57, 58
Streptomycin, 209, 210
Stress incontinence, 127
Stroke, 120, 135, 138, 140
Structural brain damage, 111
Study days, 24
Subclinical deficiencies, 121, 231
Suicide, 69, 279
Sunlight, 236, 259
Supervision, 308

SUBJECT INDEX

Surgery for bronchial carcinoma, 205
Symptomatic treatment, 50

T3, 156
T4, 156
T3 thyrotoxicosis 1, 160
Tape recordings, 14
Teaching in-depth, 16
Teaching methods, 14
Teaching programme, 11
Teaching, undergraduate, 4
Team, 313
Television, 10
Temperature regulation, 120
Therapeutics, 149
Therapeutic goal, 50
Therapy, 308
Thiamine, 239, 252
Thioridazine, 55, 56, 58
Thirst, 5
Thrombotic endocarditis, 216
Thyroid function tests, 160
Thyrotoxicosis, 159
Time telescoping, 14
"Tofranol", 59
Tongue, 253
Toxicity, digoxin, 222
Trained housekeepers, 313
Training, 4
Training, initial, 36
Training, specialist, 5
Transient cerebral ischaemia, 135, 138, 140

Transketolase, 252
Treatment of hypothyroidism, 159
Treatment, symptomatic, 50
Treatment of tuberculosis, 209, 210
Tremor, essential, 172
Tricyclic drugs, 72
Trifluoperazine, 56, 57, 58
"Tryptizol", 59
Tuberculosis, pulmonary, 204, 208
Tuberculosis, treatment, 209-210
Turner's syndrome, 161
Tybamate, 54

Undergraduate teaching, 4
Unmet needs, 247
Unsuitable housing, 37
Urethral prolapse, 126
Urinary incontinence, 123, 126

Valium, 52, 53
Valvular heart disease, 220
Ventilatory capacity, 199, 203
Vertebro-basilar insufficiency, 140
Video-tape, 14
Vincristine, 186
Violence, 69
Vitamins, 247
Vitamin A, 235
Vitamin B12, 194, 239, 253
Vitamin B complex, 236
Vitamin C, 162, 236, 237, 252, 256, 257.

Vitamin D, 162, 236, 258
Vitamin deficiencies, 247
Vitiligo, 158
Vocabulary, Crichton, 82
Voluntary effort, 277
Vulnerable groups, 262

"Welldorm", 55
Work capacity, 203

6-mercaptopurine, 187
6-thioguanine, 188